PENITENTIARY FITNESS

The Amazing Weight Loss Formula

J. Barrett Hawkins

DARK PLANET
PUBLISHING

AUTHOR'S NOTE

It is important to note that the information in this book is not intended as a substitute for the advice of your doctor and not intended to be prescriptive with reference to any specific ailment, but rather descriptive of one approach to preventive health care. Check with your physician before undertaking any of the practices contained in this book.

Author — J. Barrett Hawkins
Editor — Joyce Standish
Typesetting & Interior Design — Cris Wanzer
Exercise Illustrations — R.C. Slim
Cover Design — Cris Wanzer

© 2010 by J. Barrett Hawkins
Dark Planet Publishing

Printed in the United States of America
ISBN # 978-0-9791718-0-2
ISBN # 0-9791718-0-6
Library of Congress Control Number: 2009928186

Dark Planet Publishing books are available at special quantity discounts to use for sales promotions, premiums, or educational purposes. Please contact our Sales Department via our website:
www.JBarrettHawkins.com
— or by e-mail —
info@darkplanetpublishing.com
info@penfit.com

TABLE OF CONTENTS

AUTHOR'S NOTE 2
DEDICATIONS 4
FOREWORD...5
ACKNOWLEDGMENTS 6

Chapter 1
HOOKED ON HEALTH...7
Chapter 2
MEDICAL SCIENCE'S 20 FAT LOSS SECRETS...............................23
Chapter 3
AEROBIC TRAINING..29
Chapter 4
RESISTANCE TRAINING...34
Chapter 5
REST AND RECOVERY 41
Chapter 6
PROPER NUTRITION..44
Chapter 7
THE CONNECT WITH NATURE WEIGHT LOSS SOLUTION...............60
Chapter 8
THE POWER OF PURPOSE 70
Chapter 9
WORKOUT PLANS 81
Chapter 10
WARMING UP AND COOLING DOWN 84
Chapter 11
LOCKDOWN: THE 20-MINUTE TOTAL BODY WORKOUT................89
Chapter 12
WALK IN NATURE WORKOUTS 95
Chapter 13
PEAK PERFORMANCE TRAINING 101
Chapter 14
THE CONVICT'S LEAN AND MEAN WORKOUTS.............................109
Chapter 15
PAY IT FORWARD..120
Chapter 16
THE ILLUSTRATIONS...125

ABOUT THE AUTHOR 168
AUTHOR'S WEBSITE..169

DEDICATIONS

TO MY SON: Who inspires me to always try to do the right thing in any endeavor, and who brings a purpose to my life that drives me beyond words.

TO MY MOM: Whose love and support have enabled me to pursue goals that were otherwise unimaginable. Because of her, I started this book and because of her, I finished it.

TO BILLY DASE: Who taught me the body-weight resistance training exercises and who pushed and challenged me to achieve optimal health. Billy is a pioneer in the field of personal training – a real transformation elicitor.

TO CHARLIE GILBERTSON, JIM MOON & DANIEL DURLAND: My trainees, who offered me the gift of their trust and became my greatest teachers by allowing me to test my exercise and nutrition theories on their bodies. This book is a testament to their sacrifices and stunning trans-formations.

TO CRIS WANZER: My multi-talented manuscript consultant who shepherded this book through every phase of its development, including typing, editing, typesetting, interior design, and cover design. This book would not have been produced without her patience, guidance, and support.

FOREWORD

What does an entrepreneurial, bright young man do to keep his mind active and his body fit within the confines of a prison? What does a person with limited access to health care do to promote his body, mind and health? J. Barrett Hawkins has written a book that gives direction to anyone whose desire is to achieve optimal health.

Obviously, Barrett can neither go to the corner grocery store to pick and choose the food he needs for three square meals a day, nor can he travel to the nearest fitness supplier for the latest in exercise equipment. But necessity can be the mother of all invention, and the limitations of the prison lifestyle have given rise to a unique, back-to-basics philosophy about nutrition and exercise: This book advocates a connect-with-nature approach to nutrition. Barrett points out that man-made foods, such as cookies, chips and soda disrupt body chemistry, which in turn leads to weight gain. The author also prefers an all-natural approach to bodybuilding. Since the California prison system does not provide weights for the inmates, Barrett devised an exercise system based on pushing and pulling one's own body weight. Not surprisingly, this type of training produces a physique that is remarkably similar to that of an Olympic gymnast.

Barrett's approach to weight loss focuses on energy balance—the only medically proven method. Any physician or nutritionist will confirm if you burn more calories than you consume, you will lose weight; this is what energy balance is all about. It is that simple. It is total calories, not low carb, no fat, grapefruit, all cereal, fast one day a week or whatever the latest fad consists of. It is energy consumption minus total energy expenditure, which can be as simple as a daily time set aside for exercise, walking from the farthest space on a parking lot instead of looking for one closer. It is as simple as walking the stairs instead of taking an elevator or escalator.

Barrett doesn't have these luxuries, yet he points you in the right direction. Within the confines of a penitentiary he gives instruction to all of us who strive for health, by using up-to-date scientific research and common sense methods acquired by experience with limited resources. Read and stay fit is this doctor's advice.

Alan M. Londe, MD
Chief of Staff
Barnes Jewish West County Hospital
St. Louis, Missouri

ACKNOWLEDGMENTS

Marsha Sinetar, in her insightful book, *The Mentor's Spirit*, suggests, "The capacity to venture out to the cutting edge of new ideas creates a sense of vulnerability and every change agent needs at least one trusted colleague." Having developed the Hooked On Health program from a prison cell, I was not fortunate enough to have many trusted colleagues; however, through books, several mentors have guided my way. This work is the synergistic product of many brilliant minds. I am merely a collector and new practitioner of their transformational wisdom. I would like to acknowledge the real change agents—my health and fitness mentors—and thank them for their inspiration.

Discipline	Mentor	Primary Resource
Mind-Body Medicine	Dr. David Simon	*Training the Mind—Healing the Body*
Ayurvedic Medicine	Dr. Deepak Chopra	*Ageless Body, Timeless Mind*
Behavioral Medicine	Dr. Jon Kabat-Zinn	*Full Catastrophe Living*
Logo (Meaning) Therapy	Victor Frankl	*Man's Search for Meaning*
Psychoneuroimmunology	Daniel Goleman	*Emotional Intelligence*
Quantum Physics	Dr. Larry Dossey	*Space, Time & Medicine*
Preventive Medicine	Drs. Liponis/Hyman	*Ultraprevention*
Weight Loss	Dr. Mark Hyman	*Ultra Metabolism*
Weight Loss	Dr. Nicholas Perricone	*The Perricone Weight Loss Diet*
Nutrition	Dr. T. Colin Campbell	*The China Study*
Bodybuilding	Robert Kennedy	*The Encyclopedia of Bodybuilding*
Bodybuilding	Jeff Volek	*TNT Diet*
Kinesiology	Dr. David R. Hawkins	*Power vs. Force*
Executive Coaching	Stephen Covey	*The 7 Habits of Highly Effective People*
Personal Coaching	Cheryl Richardson	*Take Time for Your Life*
Peak Performance	Anthony Robbins	*Ultimate Power*
Psychology	Abraham Maslow	*The Farthest Reaches of Human Nature*
Inner Peace	Dr. Wayne Dyer	*10 Secrets for Success & Inner Peace*
Exercise Physiology	Dr. John Hussman	*Why the Body-for-Life Program Works*
Yoga	Gary Kraftsow	*Yoga for Wellness*
Yoga	Godfrey Devereau	*Dynamic Yoga*
Fitness Training	Bill Phillips	*Body-for-Life*
Fitness Training	Blair Whitmarsh	*Mind & Muscle*
Vision	B. Joseph Pine and James H. Gilmore	*The Experience Economy*
	Ken O'Donnell	Personal Interviews

It is also important to acknowledge Joy Thisted, a manuscript typist who took my jumbled early drafts and helped transform them into a legible manuscript.

Chapter

1

HOOKED ON HEALTH

My name is J. Barrett Hawkins. In 1987, at the age of 24, I was living the aspiring entrepreneur's dream. After failing miserably with my first three business ventures, I finally found a niche. My chain of retail clothing stores, Just Sweats, had grown from one location to 22 with annual revenues of 10 million dollars in just three years. With a growing list of franchise requests, the company was on the threshold of a national expansion. A sportswear magazine even interviewed me for an article they were writing about Just Sweats, and I boldly announced my goal of opening three hundred stores from coast to coast within five years. It was the happiest time of my life. I was in love with one of the sweetest, most gorgeous women on the planet, and my career had reached heights previously unimaginable. Little did I know it was all about to end.

Like many people who start their own business, I developed a profound emotional attachment to the company that I built. Along the way I also acquired an untamable attraction to risk. That combination proved toxic when my business partner proposed an insurance fraud that would enable me to reacquire his 45-percent ownership in Just Sweats. At that time I viewed insurance companies as corrupt, soulless entities, and faced no moral roadblock when it came to fleecing them. But something went wrong — very wrong. In the process of facilitating the fraud, my partner killed a man and I was held accountable. I was tried and convicted of conspiracy to commit murder and sentenced to twenty-five years to life in prison.[*]

---

[*] For readers interested in details of the insurance fraud, it is described in my audio book titled *The Dirty Nasty Truth,* which is available on my website: www.JBarrettHawkins.com.

The insurance fraud was presented to me by my partner as a white-collar, victimless crime. In my lifetime I have never intentionally harmed another human being. I did not intend or suspect that my business partner would commit a murder; however, that did not, in any way, minimize my responsibility for the death of a man I did not even know. My ignorance of my partner's heinous actions was deemed completely irrelevant by the law. I should have considered the possible sinister consequences of the scheme. In retrospect, I realized that my role in the fraud was pivotal — had I not been a willing participant, the murder would not have happened. I faced the unfathomable truth that I was responsible for a homicide. I could not begin to imagine the horror that the victim's family experienced, or the agony that crushed their hearts. I felt overwhelming shame and deep sorrow for the pain I had caused them, and for the embarrassment I had caused my own family. My inner turmoil led to chronic depression, nervous breakdowns, and a suicide attempt.

The only thing that sustained me through this personal nightmare was the love of my wife, Amelia, and our five-year-old son, Luke. I had told Amelia about the fraud before I committed it. Knowing that I never intended to hurt anyone, she stood by me.

During the first two years of my life sentence Amelia and Luke spent their weekends with me in the prison visiting room. As soon as my son spotted me coming through the doors, he took off at a dead sprint, leaped into my arms and fiercely hugged me. I will always remember those hugs from my little boy as the purest moments of love that I have ever felt. Amelia was the best friend I've ever had; someone who supported me during my darkest hour. Her visits were an act of extraordinary generosity. My family's love nourished my damaged soul and offered me a chance to cling to them like a newborn. Unfortunately for me, that neediness and the stigma of being a convicted felon's wife eventually drove Amelia away.

After Amelia left, I entered the most painful period of my life. A sense of hopelessness and sadness consumed every fiber of my being. From the other convicts I learned that there are more than twenty thousand prisoners in the State of California with life sentences, and no one convicted of conspiracy to commit murder had been paroled in the last seventeen years. It was a blanket policy — life meant life. I was a man with no future. My only escape from the daily oppression was exercise, but even that was lost when I severely injured my hip and ankle. With absolutely no medical care, I was laid up for a year. The inactivity led to my gaining thirty pounds of body fat and the return of an old, debilitating lower back injury. Eventually, my physical pain became as severe as my psychological pain. Thoughts of suicide returned and began to dominate my mental process.

Around this time my friend Victoria, a forensic psychologist, sent me a book by Viktor Frankl, titled *Man's Search for Meaning,* that would bring me back from the abyss. Frankl, an Austrian psychoanalyst who survived the death camps of Nazi Germany, made a significant discovery. During his three years of captivity he observed and evaluated his fellow inmates. He was intrigued by the question of what made it possible for some to survive the torture and starvation when most — 19 of every 20 — died. Those who perished had said they had no reason to live, and no longer expected anything from life. Frankl argued that they were wrong, stating, "Life's not accountable to us. We're accountable to life." And indeed it was this sense of accountability, this sense of purpose, that was the common factor in the inmates who survived. They invariably expressed that they had loved ones to return to or some important work to do or a mission to perform.[1]

Frankl developed an extraordinary insight into mankind's instinctive need for purpose. He writes: "Everyone has a specific vocation or mission in life; everyone has a concrete assignment that demands fulfillment." These insights led Frankl to develop a new type of psychotherapy called "logo (the Greek word for meaning) therapy." Logo therapy regards its assignment as that of assisting the patient to find meaning in his life. It tries to help the patient become aware of what he longs for in the depths of his heart.[2]

What I longed for was redemption; to find some way of proving to my family and to the victim's family that I am not the type of person who could knowingly be involved in the killing of a fellow human being. True, I was indirectly responsible for a man's death, but I never intended for that to happen. I am not a murderer, and I certainly did not conspire with anyone to commit a murder. Frankl's book inspired me to look within and search for a way to prove my true character.

Another author who was instrumental in helping me find my way back to wellness was Stephen Covey. His book, *The 7 Habits of Highly Effective People,* is in many ways a modern extension to

Frankl's *purpose in life therapy*. My criminal conviction, the negative publicity and the daily humiliation of the prison experience worked together to completely destroy my self-image and confidence. *7 Habits* helped me convert that negative attitude into a positive attitude by encouraging me to focus my energy on serving others, particularly those in need. This led to an epiphany. I saw that my incarceration, if viewed from a fresh perspective, could be considered a rare opportunity. Entrepreneurs are creators of concepts. Essentially what entrepreneurs do during the pre-opening stages is conduct a lot of research, then create business concepts. My realization was that I could still do what I love most in life.

In *7 Habits,* Covey writes: "Nothing has a greater, larger lasting impression upon another person than the awareness that someone has transcended suffering, has transcended circumstance and is embodying and expressing a value that inspires and enables and lifts life."[3] This one sentence led to monumental changes in my life, a desire to be the guy who transcended suffering and circumstance to create something noble. I made a conscious decision to apply my skills as a businessman toward something more significant than financial gain — by developing a company whose primary objective is to improve the quality of people's lives — and amazing things began to happen. In time, I would find meaning in a seemingly meaningless existence and in some magical way my physical and psychological wounds began to heal.

Exactly what type of business I would develop began to take shape while I was reading Dr. Deepak Chopra's classic, *Ageless Body, Timeless Mind.* The book's emphasis is on mind-body medicine. I found myself analyzing my mother's health condition. Over a three-year period she had suffered an endless series of illnesses and ailments that her doctors never properly diagnosed. This was preceded by a prolonged bout of clinical depression. A search for the cause was not difficult; in just three years she lost the three people she was closest to. First, her mother died. Next, her lifelong best friend of 40 years lost her life to cancer. Finally, her son was sent to prison with a life sentence. She was alone in the world and her depression had manifested itself in the form of physical ailments.

Chopra's book provided a concise explanation of how my mother's mental anguish led to her health problems. It also enabled me to see that her three years of suffering could have been reduced to three months with a proper mind-body diagnosis and a pro-active recovery plan. I did some research and quickly realized that, just like my mother, millions of suffering people were not getting the proper treatment. So, I decided to focus my passion for business on designing a health care facility that would fill the obvious void. In time, it became my personal mission, "my concrete assignment that demanded fulfillment."

Early on, a man named Ken O'Donnell, a high-ranking IBM executive and former *Inc Magazine* "Entrepreneur of the Year" award winner befriended me. Ken was suffering from the neurological disorder Lou Gehrig's Disease, and had a keen interest in the mind-body observations I was making. During the twilight of his life Ken became my mentor. Through letters and phone conversations we discussed a number of possibilities for a new kind of treatment center. He explained the emerging role the Internet was playing in health care and guided me through various strategies for developing a business in the New Economy. Of particular significance was something that he taught me about fund raising. Ken said that venture capitalists are attracted to business plans supported by the world's top futurists, and instructed me to study their books and reports. In one of these books, *The Experience Economy*, authors B. Joseph Pine and James H. Gilmore suggest:

> **Everyone faced with a tremendous personal loss must go through a series of experiences such as shock, depression, confusion, guilt and anger before recovery can occur. How much better can we handle these stages and more quickly be transformed from grief to normal living when someone — minister, counselor or friend — guides us, than when we are left alone. In the same way all *transformation elicitors* guide aspirants through a series of experiences.[4]**

This information made a lot of sense to me, because both my mother and I faced a tremendous personal loss. For my mother, it was the death of her own mother, her closest friend and her son's imprisonment. For me, it was the loss of my wife and son, my freedom and my self-respect. We both experienced each of these stages the authors described. However, there was a significant difference in our ability to recover. Where my mother's recovery took many years, mine actually occurred during one 12-week window of time; the primary

difference being that I was guided by various *transformation elicitors.*
Viktor Frankl and Stephen Covey guided me through a
transformation that gave my life meaning. During the same time frame
that I was making these psychological changes, I met a young convict
named Billy Dase who had just completed Bill Phillips' *Transformation Challenge*, a 12-week diet and exercise regimen that
produces amazing physiological changes. Billy encouraged me to read
Phillips' book, *Body-for-Life*, then challenged me to do the program
with him. I was 30 pounds overweight and out of shape, so I decided
to give it a try. The workout component consists of three 45-minute
sessions of high-intensity resistance training and three 20-minute
sessions of high-intensity cardiovascular exercise every week for 12
weeks. In the beginning it was grueling. My body was sore all the
time. On several occasions I wanted to quit, but Billy kept pushing and
challenging me. Peer pressure can be a powerful motivator. At week
six I started seeing results and that got me over the hump. The end of
the program coincided with my thirty-seventh birthday. I was in the
best shape of my life and actually had developed a body like one of
those guys on the cover of *Men's Health* magazine. But more
importantly, the pains in my hip, ankle and lower back were gone. The
body aches I had endured for more than three years had completely
disappeared. And so had my depression.

The latest studies from the field of psychoneuroimmunology
demonstrate that rigorous physical exercise can be a powerful weapon
in the war against depression. In his book, *Body-for-Life*, Bill Phillips
addresses this issue:

**The people who took the Transformation Challenge were
getting physically fit, and they were getting their lives back in
shape. It was, and still is, one of the most enlightening
experiences of my life. Accepting this challenge rekindled the
flame of desire for tens of thousands, and it broke down walls
that were keeping people from moving forward in all areas of
their lives.**

**Many of the men and women who accepted my challenge
reported that the program literally saved their lives. Their risk
of heart disease —the number-one killer in America today —
was drastically lowered, as well as the risk of being afflicted
with other illness, such as diabetes, cancer and osteoporosis.**

Beyond even that, the psychological and emotional changes reported by these men and women were (and are) stunning. They described off-the-chart leaps in self-confidence, self-respect, and empowerment. They discovered that taking control of their bodies broke down barriers all around them. [5]

I had the exact same experience discussed by Phillips. Even though serving a life sentence in prison, I felt good about myself and the things I was working on. My recovery from suicidal depression and chronic lower back, hip and ankle pain might never have occurred without the guidance I received from Viktor Frankl, Steven Covey, Bill Phillips, Billy Dase and Gary Kraftsow, my yoga instructor. In a very real sense, they were my *transformation elicitors*. Looking objectively at my recovery made it clear that I had unwittingly infused my system with a number of harmonizing influences within that 12-week period: strength training, aerobic training, yoga, a healthy diet, purpose in life therapy, vitamins and nutritional supplements (I was taking glucosamine sulfate, which several studies reported causes the body to produce new joint cartilage). I firmly believe the combination of these harmonizing influences created a synergistic effect, thus accelerating my return to optimal mental and physical health.

Another futurist that Ken recommended was the Institute of the Future, who predict: "By the year 2010, mental illness, particularly clinical depression, will eclipse cancer as the leading cause of disability in the United States." At first glance, this prediction seemed a bit far-fetched. But in considering how my mother's depression led to a host of other health problems, I was able to see the underlying truths. The research on depression shows that it makes other serious diseases dramatically worse. Heart disease leads a long list of illnesses that worsen with depression. People with such illnesses as cancer, arthritis, epilepsy and osteoporosis all run a higher risk of disability or premature death when clinically depressed.[6]

I had intimate knowledge of the evil that is depression, and thanks to my "health mentors," I had also gained an understanding of how to combat the problem. I saw that the process of overcoming depression, as well as being overweight or even having back problems, could be much quicker and less arduous if people have *transformation elicitors* to guide them through the changes they need to make.

In *The Experience Economy*, Pine and Gilmore predict that what is coming next is the *Transformation Economy*. They believe businesses that focus on transforming some aspect of the consumer's life will achieve market dominance. In accessing this prediction, I quickly recognized that Bill Phillips (Transformation Challenge) was a successful pioneer in the Transformation Economy. I was granted one of those moments of exceptional clarity that allows you to see things at a deeper level of meaning. I had stumbled onto something quite significant and wanted to share it with the rest of the world by designing a medical center where suffering individuals could undergo a health care transformation. I wanted to develop a *transformation center*.

From my prison cell I spent the next 10 years researching and designing an entirely new type of health care establishment called "Hooked On Health." From the beginning I saw that I had an opportunity that businessmen in the "real world" could only dream of: An infinite amount of time to conduct research and create. For years all I did was read and apply what I learned to the task at hand. I read hundreds of books by cutting-edge physicians and innovative entrepreneurs, and integrated their wisdom into the Hooked On Health business plan.

One of the best books I discovered on creating health is *Ultraprevention,* by Dr. Mark Liponis and Dr. Mark Hyman. Their medical model is information based; a system of treatment derived from the scientific study of health. These doctors took the time to keep up with research studies and incorporate the newest discoveries.[7]

I followed their lead, and medical research studies became the foundation upon which Hooked On Health was built. The treatment model is based on the principles of mind-body medicine, which encourages patients to get in touch with their purpose in life and pursue peak physical conditioning as the ultimate form of prevention. These objectives will be facilitated through an evolutionary concept — Self-Care Mentorship — in which doctors and other health care professionals will utilize a series of seminars, courses and workshops to teach their patients methods of extreme self-care. The mentorship forum will be combined with lifestyle coaching and personal-fitness training sessions with the expectation that the cross-fertilization will guide people to optimal health. These core competencies, offered in a cost-effective mini-group formula and dynamically connected as 12-week transformation programs, will serve as the foundation for *Pro-*

Active Health Care, a new, action-based paradigm in behavioral medicine.

During the period of time that I was designing Hooked On Health, I met a sixty-eight-year-old, retired fireman named Charlie who was in prison for killing a gang member who had raped his fourteen-year-old daughter. Charlie was sentenced to sixteen years for manslaughter. The thought of dying in prison led to extreme depression and an overwhelming sense of guilt. Charlie was a father of six and a devoted husband. The entire incident had devastated his wife and he also shouldered the burden of her pain. Charlie is a good man. He had never previously broken the law and spent most of his adult life working to better his community. I wanted to help and offered to guide him through the transformation program I had learned from Billy. Charlie had not exercised in ten years and initially was not receptive to the prospect of intense training. However, I was successful in persuading him to read *Ageless Body, Timeless Mind.* One entire section of the book studies centenarians (individuals who live for more than one hundred years) and emphasized regular exercise as a critical component in longevity. Charlie saw an opportunity to outlive his sentence and return to his family.

So, he agreed to let me train him. The first few weeks were brutal. He was so sore he could not even get out of bed on a number of occasions. I motivated him by preaching that if he got in top physical condition, he would someday get to go home. Charlie stuck with it and by the end of the program was a new man. Not only did his body look like that of a professional athlete, but also his depression completely disappeared. He became optimistic about his future, enrolling in a Bible College and making plans to become a minister.

I vividly recall a day when he took off his shirt, flexed a brilliantly sculptured double bicep and said to me, "Hey kid, take a look at your handiwork." It warmed my heart to see the old rooster strut. After our workouts he often said, "I feel so good, thanks to you." Knowing that I was instrumental in helping Charlie find his way back to health and happiness was rewarding. Every time he thanked me, I was reminded of how important my Hooked On Health mission is and how grateful I am to have discovered the meaning of my own life.

Charlie really opened my eyes to the role a transformation center could play in longevity, anti-aging and the quality of a senior citizen's life. In the beginning, Charlie could not do a single pull-up. By the end of the program he could bring maximum intensity to every exercise for a full forty-five-minute workout. I even had him doing wind sprints three days a week. The effect this had on his self-esteem and sense of vitality was stunning. Charlie felt younger, stronger and more in control of his life. At the age of sixty-eight he had transformed his body from that of a flabby old man to a physique every bit as muscular and sculptured as that of a bodybuilder. Every morning he looked in the mirror and felt good about himself, which certainly played a major role in his ability to overcome depression.

Charlie's impressive physique and newfound physical prowess quickly became the talk of the prison yard. He was running circles around convicts half his age. Word got around, and it was not long before another man, Jim, asked me to train him. Jim was forty-seven years of age and nearly a hundred pounds overweight. From my research, I knew that 65 percent of the American population was overweight and that excess fat leads to an array of other health problems including heart disease, diabetes, stroke, high blood pressure, and certain types of cancer. I wanted Hooked On Health to offer fat-loss transformation programs, so this was a challenge I could not refuse. I decided I would learn everything there was to know about losing weight and dedicated myself to helping Jim overcome his obesity.

As Jim and I got to know one another, I learned that he was also an entrepreneur. He had owned a small business and had experience in franchising. He also had an addiction to methamphetamine and easy money. This was his third time in prison as a result of selling drugs, and he was determined to break the pattern. He spent two years in a prison drug rehabilitation program called Amity and got straight for the first time in his adult life. Jim confided in me his desire to work with addicts when he got out.

I shared my dream of opening Hooked On Health, and he convinced me that the transformation center should offer programs for drug abusers. Jim felt that the training regimen through which I was guiding him (exercise, diet and purpose in life therapy) complemented the group therapy he was getting with Amity and had been instrumental in helping him overcome his addiction. He was involved in a training course to become an Amity counselor and had a wealth of knowledge about fighting drug abuse. I learned that 75 percent of the men in prison had committed crimes that were drug-related.

Dr. Chopra describes drug abuse as a lack of exultation; meaning that something is missing from a person's life and they are using drugs to fill the void. According to mind-body medicine the cure is to help users get in touch with their purpose in life, to replace the high of the drugs with the exultation of *meaning;* I explained this to Jim and he agreed with me wholeheartedly. Jim has three children and he said that fulfilling his responsibilities as a father is what gave his life meaning and purpose; he started developing a plan to enable him to do just that when he got out. At the same time he was becoming involved in assisting me with Hooked On Health. We worked on mock-up transformation programs and eventually designed a drug rehab program that combined purpose in life therapy, group therapy and intense physical training.

Over time I came to believe that Jim could help me get the business off the ground. During our workouts we discussed the intricacies of the business plan and worked on his presentation. Jim worked out hard and maintained strong discipline on his diet. In the course of six months he took eleven inches off a flabby waistline and put his body in peak physical condition. His transformation was incredible both physically and psychologically. By the time of his release I was confident that he was the right person to represent my vision.

Shortly after Jim went home, I received the following letter from him, which I would like to share with you. In the letter he refers to me as "Cap," which is short for Captain, and is in reference to my work as a yacht skipper many years ago.

My Friend "Cap,"

As I stated in the letter to my brother, just saying goodbye seemed to leave a void. Sometimes in parting important thoughts and emotions are easier expressed when written, which is why I felt compelled to write this to you.

Although our time together has been relatively short, I feel that the time spent had essential characteristics of high merit. "Quality," know it or not, you were a true inspiration. Thanks to you, I look and feel like a new man. Thank you for guiding me through my transformation. You truly are a "Transformation Elicitor."

As the Captain of my sea into tomorrow, I give you a true

heartfelt thanks for allowing me to be your first mate. Know that I
will give 110% to our quest. I'm excited to be a part of your vision.
And I hope you know I share in it as well.

   So my mentor, my Captain, my friend — this is not a
goodbye, but it is a letter of hope and aspiration for you. Know
that you have made a great and wonderful change in my life.
Keep doing the things that you do, know that God will bless you
sooner than you can imagine.

   With love,
   Your Friend and First Mate, Jim

   The letter unleashed a flood of emotion and I could not control
the tears that ran down my face. I had worked so hard for so many
years, but rarely had there been a sign that it had been worth the effort.
But, like Charlie before him, Jim's transformation reminded me of how
important this work is and of the impact Hooked On Health will have
in people's lives.

   Two weeks after Jim got out, he met with a San Diego attorney
whom he had known for years. The two men spent hours going over
every detail of the business plan. The attorney loved the concept and
said he knew some investors in Las Vegas who might be interested in
funding the business. Unfortunately, Jim never got the opportunity to
meet with them because of the 9-11 terrorist attack on Manhattan's
Twin Towers. The economy went south, Vegas in particular. The
investors the lawyer had lined up were no longer looking at any new
deals, and rightfully so. It was the absolute worst time to open a new
business. Jim and I joined the rest of the country in a national state of
depression.

   I spent the first couple of months following 9-11 feeling sorry
for myself. The media naysayers were predicting a prolonged
recession and for a period of time I lost sight of my vision. When
Hooked On Health was put on an indefinite back burner, my sense of
purpose vanished. Like a rudderless ship caught in a rip tide, I drifted
into the shadowy prison underworld. The gray walls, the barbed wire,
guards barking out orders, horrendous people with whom I had to deal
on a daily basis, my own lack of exultation — the prison world soon
became unbearable.

   I desperately wanted to connect with people in the "real world"
who shared my dream of developing a medical center, where

individuals in need could transform their lives. But fear of rejection had wounded me. I had been convicted of an intolerable crime and could not conceive of a way to overcome my status of "life prisoner." Self-pity and procrastination became my maladies, destroying my inner confidence and willingness to take chances. My dream was dying because I saw myself as Americans view all convicted felons — a piece of garbage discarded by society. The bad thoughts returned in abundance. At this crossroads in my life all forms of escapism looked appealing, and I could not conceive of a way to change that.

Intuitively, my mother seemed to know how to pull me out of the doldrums. On Thanksgiving Day she suggested that I write a health and fitness book detailing the transformation program through which I had guided Charlie and Jim. A convict's approach to fitness! She said that there was nothing like it. And she was correct — convicts use training methods of which most people have never even heard. I liked the idea immediately because it would enable me to recapture my focus on serving others.

The workout program I learned from Billy had evolved into something truly unique. Even though conceived on the principles of *Body-for-Life*, the program was really quite different. Since the California prison system does not allow the inmates to use weights, Billy found a way to stimulate every muscle group through a rather ingenious high-intensity, body-weight resistance training regimen. By body-weight resistance I mean pull-up and push-up type exercises. Over time, I have interviewed other convicts who developed extraordinary physiques and incorporated their methods. I have also added yoga, some Pilates and a cardiovascular regimen used by world-class athletes. These elements, combined with the insights gained from my decade-long study of nutrition and mind-body medicine, came together to form a peak athletic performance and optimal health transformation program that I call *Hooked On Health*.

In my personal opinion, Olympic gymnasts and sprinters (both male and female) have the most beautiful physiques on the planet. Thus, I designed the exercise component of the transformation program to emulate their training methods. When you combine the athletic grace of gymnastics (pushing and pulling one's own bodyweight) with the explosiveness of all-out sprinting, the results are extraordinary: powerful, multifunctional muscles with extremely sharp lines of definition. The *Hooked On Health* program aspires to help you build a beautiful body, but perhaps more importantly, the system is designed to help you live a longer, healthier life. It will also drastically lower your risk of many diseases, including heart disease, cancer, diabetes, osteoporosis and arthritis. It will strengthen your heart, your cardiovascular system, your immune system, and increase your balance, flexibility and coordination. Thus, peak athletic performance becomes the ultimate form of disease and injury prevention.

Since I am not a doctor or even a certified personal fitness trainer, I decided to base the program's recommendations on research studies conducted at the world's top medical schools and universities. As previously mentioned, medical research studies were the foundation upon which the transformation center business concept was built. "The treatment model was derived from the scientific study of health and incorporated the newest discoveries."[7] Research studies provide a fascinating look at the inner-workings of the human body and at the same time can inspire us to make changes that will improve the quality of our own lives. These studies provide the basic framework of the *Hooked On Health* system.

The research studies also motivated me to develop an exciting new weight loss solution. Over the last 10 years I have read hundreds of published studies on the subject of weight loss, and I began to see patterns within the information. One medical school would discover that a particular food, nutritional supplement or type of exercise would produce dramatic results; then another research facility would analyze the same stimulus and confirm its effectiveness for weight loss. These findings inspired me to cross-reference and synthesize all of the relevant information, and what emerged was *The Amazing Weight Loss Formula.* This formula evolved from a simple and logical insight: When a person does everything that modern science says they should do to lose weight, then they will have the best possible results.

The research revealed that developing muscle mass through high-intensity resistance training was by far the most significant factor in weight loss. When you add muscle, your metabolism speeds up. The word "metabolism" describes the body's ability to burn calories (energy) on an ongoing basis. Ultimately, weight loss comes down to energy balance: When you burn more energy through your daily activities and maintaining your body mass than you consume through your diet, your body is forced to tap into its back-up energy supply — its fat stores.[8]

The daily maintenance of one pound of muscle requires 70 times more calories than one pound of fat.[9] That's a dramatic finding and is why high-intensity resistance training is so important for people who want to lose weight. It is also why a convict's approach to weight loss could be revolutionary. Convicts train at off-the-chart levels of intensity and that leads to extraordinary results.

It is also important to note that this result was exactly the same for women. In fact, women will find body-weight resistance training to be an ideal way to burn fat, trim their tummy and shape their derriere. Many women refuse to lift weights because they fear becoming too muscular, or don't want to exercise at a gym with a bunch of guys staring at them. Getting too muscular is a misconception created by the appearance of female bodybuilders, most of whom take steroids. Normal women simply do not have enough testosterone to develop big muscles.[10] Going to a gym is also a non-issue because the *Hooked On Health* workouts do not require any equipment. Body-weight resistance training can be done in the park, at the beach, or even in one's own backyard. By exercising outdoors we gain the added benefit of connecting with nature. Sunshine, fresh air and beautiful scenery nourish the body, mind and soul.

A look ahead: Chapter 2 lists medical science's top twenty fat-loss secrets. Chapter 3 suggests that you get your aerobic training by engaging in high-intensity sports and other activities that you enjoy. Chapter 4 explains exactly how muscles develop and why it is so important for weight loss. Chapter 5 emphasizes the need for rest and provides techniques that will help you sleep better and recover faster. Chapter 6 breaks down the science of nutrition in terms that are easy to understand. Chapter 7 takes that nutrition information and shows you how to create your own meal plans.

The remaining sections of the book focus primarily on personal motivation and the various workout plans. Chapter 8 relates the story of Daniel Durland, a young man who lost 110 pounds of body fat in five months using the *Hooked On Health* system and discusses the virtues of infusing your life (and workouts) with purpose. Chapter 9 matches individual objectives with specific workout plans. Chapter 10 explains the importance of warming up before a training session and cooling down afterward. Chapter 11, the 20-Minute Total Body Workout, is designed for busy, time-starved individuals. Chapters 12 and 13 detail exercise routines that will help you develop a body similar to that of an Olympic gymnast. Chapter 14 discusses the most advanced workouts for both muscle development and fat loss. Chapter 15 offers a preview of my next book, *Principles of Grace: The Teachings of the Medicine Man*. And finally, Chapter 16 provides illustrations and step-by-step instructions for each of the exercises. Most of the chapters are brief and concise, some only a few pages, but all are power-packed with the knowledge you will need to achieve optimal health and to develop your best body.

2

MEDICAL SCIENCE'S 20 FAT LOSS SECRETS

In the United States, 65 percent of the adult population is overweight.[1] Four hundred thousand Americans die each year from health problems directly related to being overweight.[2] Not surprisingly, two landmark research studies reported by *USA Today's* Nanci Hellmich reveal that maintaining a healthy weight is a major factor in human longevity.

- In a study published in the prestigious *Journal of the American Medical Association,* researchers from Johns Hopkins Medical School concluded that a severely obese (50 or more pounds overweight) white man would lose 13 years of life expectancy and a similar black man would lose 20 years.[3]

- A study published in the *Annals of Internal Medicine* examined data from the renowned Framingham Heart Study and found that moderate obesity (30-50 pounds overweight) reduced a person's lifespan by seven years; and that even carrying an extra 10 to 30 pounds could shorten one's life by about three years.[4]

Excess fat imposes a significant burden on internal organs and generates inflammatory molecules called "free radicals" that damage cells, increasing the risk of heart disease and cancer; the two biggest causes of death for human beings. Obesity is also the primary cause of Type-2 diabetes, which can lead to blindness, kidney failure, aneurysms, neuropathy and amputation of limbs.

The good news is that in most cases these conditions are reversible — if the sufferer loses the toxic body fat. The better news is that losing body fat is not as difficult as most people think. In this brief chapter I have accumulated medical science's top 20 fat-loss secrets, each of which works. When you apply all 20 secrets over a 12-week period of time, it creates a synergy within the body that accelerates fat burning exponentially.

#20 Sleep eight hours every night
A survey of 87,000 United States adults by the Centers for Disease Control and Prevention showed that people who slept seven to eight hours a night had significantly lower obesity rates when compared to people who slept less than six hours a night. Sleep deprivation increases a hormone called ghrelin, which increases appetite. It also reduces leptin, a hormone that normally suppresses appetite.[5]

#19 Practice portion control
From the Big Gulp to the Double Whopper to a jumbo-sized order of French fries, the U.S. has become a "super-sized" nation. According to a study published in the *Journal of the American Medical Association (JAMA)*, the average American's total daily calorie intake has risen from 1850 to 2150 over the past twenty years, due primarily to increased portion sizes.[6] These over-sized portions are a big part of the obesity problem, because whatever food the body does not need for energy and cell regeneration, it stores as fat. Our hunter/gatherer ancestors had very adaptive metabolisms designed to "store" excess calories to fuel their bodies during times of famine; this is part of our genetic structure.[7] Instead of eating large super-sized meals, someone who wants to shed fat should…

#18 Eat five to six small meals every day
When you eat large meals the body uses only what it needs and stores the rest in the form of fat for times of famine. When your body goes too long without a meal it perceives a famine and releases enzymes and hormones that "protect" fat stores.[8] By eating small, frequent meals, you are able to maintain a steady flow of nutrients and energy, stabilize your moods and increase "thermogenesis." The thermic response to food relates to the calories your body burns, as you digest your food. More calories burned equals more fat loss.

#17 Reduce stress
Stress causes the body to release a hormone called "cortisol" which triggers a strong craving for high-carbohydrate snacks. Cortisol also causes the breakdown of muscle tissue and inhibits glucose (food) from getting into the cells, causing a further wasting of muscle.[9]

#16   Drink green tea instead of coffee
A study conducted at the University of Geneva (France) found that men given green tea extract three times a day increased their metabolic rate and burned more fat for fuel during exercise.[10] Coffee, on the other hand, causes a rise in cortisol levels that can last up to 12 hours.

#15   Give up fried foods completely
Researchers are finding that fried foods such as potato chips and French fries disrupt the signals between the hormone leptin and the brain, causing you to gain fat much faster than any other type of food. Leptin is a hormone responsible for cutting appetite and sending the "full" signal to the brain. Fried foods also drastically raise your cholesterol levels, clog your arteries and can cause you to feel sluggish.

#14   No carbs after dinner
The body converts carbohydrates into glucose, which is our primary energy source, but when glycogen stores are full, any extra carbs will be stored as fat. Since activity levels decrease for most people after dinner, any additional carbs will be deposited in the stomach or "love handle" area of your body. If you get hungry late in the evening, then I suggest you . . .

#13   Eat more protein
The latest medical research indicates that a high protein diet is effective for weight loss.[11] The reasons for this effectiveness include: (1) a higher thermic response — the body burns about 30 percent of each protein calorie during digestion versus only eight percent for carbs and two percent for fats; (2) increased satiety — the slower rate of digestion results in the feeling of hunger being abated for a longer period of time; (3) increased growth hormone secretion — a hormone that plays a major role in muscle development and fat loss.

#12   Supplement with whey protein
Protein is comprised of 20 building blocks called amino acids. Whey protein contains the highest content (25 percent) of branch-chain amino acids (BCAA's) of any single protein source. According to researchers this BCAA content is important for fat loss. In one study,[12]

wrestlers who combined BCAA's with a low-calorie nutrition plan lost 34 percent more abdominal fat compared to others who followed the same diet but did not use the BCAA's. Researchers have also found that whey protein strengthens the immune system.

#11   Eat foods that are low in energy density
In a study developed at Pennsylvania State University, researchers discovered that women who consumed foods with a low energy density consumed fewer calories than when they ate foods with a higher energy density.[13] The term "energy density" refers to a food's calorie content. Foods found in nature — fruits, vegetables, nuts, whole grains —are low in energy density. These foods are also high in nutrient density, thus promoting satiety on fewer calories.

#10   Eat a healthy, balanced breakfast every day
Breakfast is the most important meal of the day…if your goal is to lose weight. A study involving 3,000 individuals who lost an average of 70 pounds and kept it off for six years ate breakfast regularly, compared to only four percent who skipped breakfast.[14] A balanced breakfast, including a portion of lean protein (eggs), a portion of whole grain (oatmeal), and a piece of fruit will "set" your metabolism for the day and reduce unnecessary hunger cravings.

#9   Give up soft drinks completely
Soda and juice drinks that are not 100 percent juice are quite possibly the most fattening things on the planet. A 20-oz. bottle of Coke contains 250 calories. If you drink one bottle a day every day for a year, you will gain 26 pounds of body fat. Sugary drinks also contain large amounts of high-fructose corn syrup. As with fried foods, medical research indicates that this substance causes you to gain fat faster than other food sources. If you are looking for an alternative beverage, I recommend that you…

#8   Drink more water
According to a study reported in *Muscle & Fitness* magazine, a person can raise their resting metabolic rate by drinking eight 8-ounce glasses of water a day. The researchers measured the metabolisms of 14 men and women before and after they drank 16 ounces of water. Within 10 minutes their metabolisms began to rise. After 40 minutes, the test

subjects' average calorie-burning rate was 30 percent higher, and it remained elevated for more than an hour.[15] It is also worth noting that water does not contain any calories.

#7   Eat more foods that are naturally rich in water
Water-rich foods means more veggies — a lot more. Most vegetables are 90-95 percent water. One of the most amazing benefits of vegetables is that they are extremely low in calories, so you can eat a lot of them without worrying about weight gain. Other low-calorie, water-based foods include non-tropical fruit and soups.

#6   Choose fish instead of beef
Beef is high in saturated fat, which leads to weight gain and heart disease. Fish (particularly salmon, sardines, tuna and mackerel) are high in omega three fatty acids, which promote weight loss by increasing insulin sensitivity and fat burning during exercise. Fish also increases good HDL cholesterol that is important for fighting heart disease.[16]

#5   Trade TV time for evening walks
According to an Auburn University study, men who viewed TV more than three hours a day were twice as likely to be obese as those who watched less than one hour a day.[17] Inactivity leads to weight gain, but you can reverse this trend by trading in your TV and computer time for long evening walks or other outdoor activities that you enjoy.

#4   Eat more foods with fiber
Foods that are rich in fiber — whole grains, beans, nuts, seeds, fruits and vegetables — are important for weight loss. Fiber promotes satiety because it absorbs water and expands in the stomach; this in turn sends a "full" signal to the brain. A diet high in fiber reduces obesity, high blood pressure and other risk factors in heart disease. Fiber also lowers levels of the hormone insulin, which is important because once energy stores are full, insulin begins to feed fat cells.[18]

#3   Create a caloric deficit
This suggestion means that you simply need to burn more calories than you consume. The best way to do this is to make a conscious effort to stay active. Take the stairs in lieu of the elevator. Instead of reading a

book, get books on tape and listen to them while taking a brisk walk. And above all, turn off the TV or computer and get your entertainment outdoors by rollerblading, jumping on a trampoline, playing softball or engaging in some type of activity you enjoy.

#2   Eat slowly and consciously

According to ayurveda — the world's oldest known system of medicine — you can change your level of satiety, which means "level of satisfaction," by practicing eating awareness.[19] In America's fast-paced, multi-tasking society, people often conduct business, read, or even watch TV while eating a meal. This has a negative effect on their satiety. Eating is meant to be a pleasurable experience. Try eating in silence, chewing your food slowly and consciously focusing your mental attention on savoring every bite. You will be amazed at how you can derive more satisfaction while actually eating less.

#1   Change your resting metabolic rate

Your resting metabolic rate describes the speed with which your body uses energy on an ongoing basis. The faster your resting metabolic rate is, the more efficiently your body burns fat. When you perform high-intensity resistance training exercises, you develop more muscle mass and your resting metabolic rate increases. When you perform high-intensity cardiovascular exercises, your heart and lungs get stronger and your resting metabolic rate increases. When you eat small, frequent, high-protein meals, your thermic response is higher and your resting metabolic rate increases. When you give your body proper rest and recovery, cells regenerate and your resting metabolic rate increases. And when you combine these four elements, you have the foundation for the ultimate peak performance and weight loss transformation program—*Penitentiary Fitness*. Read the upcoming chapters and learn how to raise your metabolism and develop your best body.

Chapter

3

AEROBIC TRAINING

This section begins with an explanation of what your metabolism is and how it works. Your diet provides the essential components of metabolism. If you look up the word "calorie" in the dictionary, you'll see that it is defined as a unit of energy; and the word "metabolism" describes your body's ability to burn energy on an ongoing basis.

During digestion, enzymes split proteins into amino acids, fats into fatty acids, and carbohydrates into blood sugar (or glucose). At this time, the body releases a hormone called insulin, which is a carrier molecule. Insulin then transports these compounds into the cells via the bloodstream. Inside of each cell there are mini power plants called the mitochondria that draw oxygen from the bloodstream to burn blood sugar and produce ATP (adenosine triphosphate) — energy.[1]

In the same way that every car has a different rate of energy efficiency, every human being burns energy at a different rate. The mitochondria is the key to determining your metabolic rate. Dr. Mark Hyman, author of the book *Ultrametabolism,* explains:

> **Mitochondria are the parts of the cells that combine the calories you consume with oxygen and turn this mixture into energy, used to run everything in your body. A single cell may have anywhere from 200-2,000 mitochondria. Cells that work hard such as those in the heart, liver, or muscle, contain the greatest number.**
>
> **The rate at which your mitochondria transform food and oxygen into energy is called your metabolic rate, and it is determined by two factors: the number of mitochondria you have and how effectively they burn oxygen and calories.[2]**

Aerobic exercise, particularly high-intensity interval training, enables this system to function more effectively. With high-intensity interval training you use bursts of intensity to raise your heart rate in intervals. For example, in a running workout you could alternate walking, jogging, and sprinting. High-intensity interval training will raise your metabolism and your fat burning potential. Again, I refer to Hyman for insight:

> **This type of training helps the body become more efficient at taking in oxygen, which in turn makes the muscle cells produce more mitochondria and makes the mitochondria you have more efficient.**

> **By increasing the number and function of the mitochondria in your body, you increase your ability to burn calories at rest; hence, you increase the number of calories burned even while you sit at your computer checking e-mail or sleep.**[3]

In a study conducted at Canada's Laval University[4] researchers compared the traditional slow-go aerobics (jogging) with high-intensity interval training. The jogging group trained for more weeks (20 versus 15), used longer exercise sessions (45 minutes versus 30), worked out more frequently (90 workouts versus 60) and burned twice as many calories during their workouts. However, *the high-intensity interval training group burned nine times more body fat.* The reason for these results, says researchers, is that the interval training transformed the test subjects' metabolisms, enabling them to burn calories at a greater rate 24-hours a day.

In addition to raising your metabolic rate, high-intensity interval training will also dramatically lower your risk for heart disease. Heart attacks occur because the arteries narrow as the result of plaque buildup. High-intensity interval training increases the volume of blood the heart is forced to pump and rushes the blood through the arteries at a greater rate. That strengthens the heart, widens the arteries and reduces the damaging effects of triglycerides (the fats that develop into plaque). If you want to achieve optimal health, it is imperative that you do high-intensity aerobics. Additionally, it is important for you to enjoy your workouts.

Another interesting study conducted in Sweden and published in the *British Medical Journal* focused on using behavior modification to reduce the risk factors in heart disease, and succinctly illustrates this point. In the study one group of patients were instructed to stop smoking, exercise, lose weight, change their eating habits and lower their cholesterol. The control group was not given any lifestyle intervention instructions. The researchers assumed that the first group would experience a lower incidence of heart disease, but they were wrong. The group that participated in the behavior modification had a significantly *higher* mortality rate. In accessing the results the editor stated, "The hassle factor or stress that was induced by wanting to change the risk factors was responsible for the even higher mortality in people who had these interventions." The individuals in this study were told that if they did not lose weight and lower their cholesterol they would have a heart attack.[5] They tried to motivate the individuals through fear. What the researchers did not know and what mind-body medicine is now teaching us is that fear creates a negative biological response that weakens our systems.

It is my belief that there is a much better way to motivate people to exercise, and that's by making it fun. For this reason, I recommend that you initially get your cardiovascular exercise by playing sports or engaging in activities that you truly enjoy. In fact, the enjoyment itself will have a positive influence on your physiology; it takes the work out of "workouts." Following is a brief listing of high-intensity interval training activities for your consideration.

Aerobic Training Activities

Boxing	Racquetball	Dancing	Kayaking
Soccer	Squash	Roller Blading	Mt. Bike Riding
Basketball	Handball	Swimming	Tennis
Flag Football	Downhill Skiing	Cycling	Ice Skating
2 on 2 Volleyball	Rock Climbing	Rowing	Skipping Rope

Swimming is probably the best way to exercise your cardio-vascular system, because unlike most land-based activities, swimming is gentle on the joints. If you do not swim, then you should vary your activities. If you do the same exercise over and over again, the repetitive stress may lead to osteoarthritis later in life; this is another lesson that I had to learn the hard way. During the first five years of my incarceration, I played basketball for two to three hours a day, every day, on a concrete surface. The constant pounding damaged all of my lower body joints: ankles, knees and hips.

I am now 46 years old, and in the seven years since Billy guided me through my transformation, I have re-injured my hips and lower back several times playing basketball. Even though I regret hurting myself, the injuries brought great insight into the human condition. One important thing I learned is that if a part of your body cannot handle a stress that is being placed upon it, that part will recruit neighboring muscles to pick up the slack. My hip injury caused my lower back muscles to overcompensate and in the process, the lower back was also hurt. Another important lesson I learned is that human beings are creatures of habit, and habits are hard to break. As you might expect, prison basketball is a violent sport; yet in spite of the dysfunctional characters with whom I had to deal and the fact that my condition was so severe that I could not even walk when I re-injured my lower back, I returned to the court as soon as the injury healed. The reason I was unwilling to break this habit is because I was doing something that I truly love, something I did when I was a free man. During those precious moments playing basketball, I did not have to acknowledge my incarceration. Of course, now I regret my poor decisions. The last time I re-injured the hip and lower back, it took six months before I was able to walk without pain. I have been rehabbing it now for an additional six months and still cannot run without experiencing extreme lower back pain. I fear that I may have caused a permanent disability.

If you get nothing else from this book, please learn this one thing: If you want to know what the state of your health will be in 20 years, all you have to do is look at how you are treating your body today. If you abuse your liver with alcohol, your lungs with cigarettes, your heart with a poor diet, or even your joints through repetitive stress, you will pay for it later in life.

During the six months I was laid up, I regained most of the fat I had lost. When capable of exercising again, I had to get rid of the fat without the high-intensity aerobics; that was far more difficult. You really do need all four elements — high-intensity aerobics, high-intensity resistance training, proper nutrition and rest — to burn fat optimally. If you are physically unable to do high-intensity aerobic activities, then try speed walking. I currently speed walk for an hour every day, and to my surprise, it always wears me out. The key is to walk fast enough to break out in a sweat. You can even incorporate some skipping, high stepping or push-up intervals to elevate your heart rate. If I again had a lot of weight to lose, I'd do the high-intensity aerobic exercises in the morning *and* add an hour of speed walking in the evening (as opposed to watching TV) to burn extra calories.

This chapter ends with another lesson I learned from the basketball court: Limit all cardio workouts to one hour, if your goal is to develop a muscular body. A lot of the guys with whom I played basketball also did resistance training, but could not add any muscle mass; when studying exercise physiology, I discovered the reason. An hour of high-intensity exercise activities will completely deplete glycogen (fuel) stores. If you continue to exercise at this point, the body becomes catabolic, meaning that it feeds off itself by breaking down muscle tissue to fuel the activity. This is the reason marathon runners often look emaciated and you see football players drinking Gatorade during the timeouts. The sports drink becomes a secondary source of fuel that can preserve muscle tissue.

Chapter

4

RESISTANCE TRAINING

High-intensity resistance training enables both men and women to develop more muscle mass, which in turn raises the resting metabolic rate. Muscle requires 70 times more calories than fat for daily maintenance.[1] For every pound of lean muscle gained, the body burns approximately 50 additional calories every day just maintaining itself. It is a simple formula: Additional muscle speeds up your metabolism and turns your body into a more efficient fat-burning system.

The human body is explicitly designed to adapt to stress, and high-intensity resistance training "stresses" your muscle fibers. The muscle adapts by getting bigger and stronger so it will be prepared to tolerate that stress if encountered in the future. High-intensity resistance training actually causes microscopic tears in the muscle fibers. Muscle growth occurs when the tear is repaired through a combination of rest and proper nutrition. This treatment also revs up your metabolism, because your body will burn calories and fat during sleep as it repairs the micro-tears.

Your muscles have two types of fibers: slow-twitch fibers, which are used during endurance activities; and fast-twitch fibers, which are used during explosive movements such as sprinting or lifting heavy weights. The fast-twitch fibers are important for developing strength and the neurological pathways required to engage the maximum number of motor units. They are stimulated through heavy resistance training; exercises in the 1- 6 repetition range. Lighter resistance training exercises in the 6 -12 repetition range tax the slow-twitch fibers, which are essential for growth and fat burning. The *Hooked On Health* training system is laid out in six completely separate phases designed to progressively stimulate all muscle fibers to ensure optimal growth and performance.

The Intensity Factor

The intensity of your exercise is one of the most important factors in muscle development and fat loss. But exactly what is intensity? In his "The Romano Factor" column, *Muscular Development* magazine's John Romano provides the perfect description:

> Cultivated from within successful bodybuilders, passion cannot be bought from a supplement shop or drugstore. It is not found in a pill, powder or syringe. It's simply an exhaustive testament of a trainee's ability to find inner courage, character, and determination.[2]

Intensity is passion, enthusiasm, and inner determination. This is exactly why Phase 1 begins by advising you to choose an activity that you truly enjoy for the high-intensity cardiovascular exercise. In sports such as basketball or tennis you may go all out on offense, then in a matter of seconds you must tap into some hidden reservoir for more energy as you transition to defense. The passion you bring to play enables you to *push your body beyond apparent limits;* that is intensity.

Your body has two primary energy systems, aerobic and anaerobic. During moderate intensity exercises, such as jogging, the body relies upon the aerobic energy system. When the intensity of the exercise requires more energy than what can be burned with the oxygen you are breathing, your body kicks into a higher gear called anaerobic glycolysis. This is the system that must be trained to attain fast results.[3] As the body activates the anaerobic system it simultaneously begins to release endorphins. This wonder drug in turn relieves stress and makes you feel really, really good. My goal during the first four weeks of the transformation program is to turn you into an endorphin junkie, to get you Hooked On Health. Once you get a taste of what optimal health feels like, I'm certain you will want more of it and eventually will bring that same passion, that same intensity to your resistance training workouts.

With resistance training it is also necessary to push your body beyond apparent limits. One of the methods used to achieve optimal results is training to failure. This technique is particularly effective at creating micro-tears in a large number of muscle fibers. Bear in mind that training to failure causes an incredible shock to the system and can lead to injury when your body is out of shape. Therefore, beginners will not use this method until week five.

Another technique you will be using to crank up the intensity is forced repetitions where your training partner will help you to push out reps beyond failure. Forced reps are utilized during Phase 3 of the workout plan.

Proper Form

When performing the body-weight resistance training exercises, proper form is paramount to achieving the desired results and avoiding injury. For this reason, Phase 1 begins with the most basic exercises. Whenever a new exercise is introduced, you must master the technique before doing maximum intensity sets. For best results, you will want to achieve powerful muscle contraction. For example, when you are performing the classic push-up, you should keep your mind focused on the muscles you are training. During the negative (lowering) motion you will keep tension on the muscle by moving slowing and deliberately. On the positive (rising) motion you will contract and squeeze the muscle at the top. This process of moving slowly to keep tension on the muscle and squeezing to contract the muscle is what causes the micro-tears in the muscle fiber.

Principles of Adaptation

As mentioned, the human body is explicitly designed to adapt to stress, and high-intensity resistance training is a form of stress. Therefore, if you give your body the same workouts over and over again, it will become very efficient at those workouts and the need to adapt will eventually disappear. Exercises that initially created micro-tears in the muscle fibers will not be intense enough to elicit ongoing changes.[4] As the muscle adapts, it becomes stronger and fewer fibers are needed to do familiar exercises. As a result, you can hit plateaus and stop making progress.

Since I am writing a fitness book, I attentively observe other people while they are working out. What I see most often is them doing the same workout over and over again. In many cases, success leads to failure. People find a routine that works and blindly do the same exercises in the same order with the exact same number of repetitions, thinking (wrongly) that the workout will continue to deliver the same results.

A perfect example of this is my friend Mike. He has been doing the same workouts for five years. He chooses the most difficult exercises, performs each of them with perfect form, and brings an intensity level that would do *Arnold* proud. Mike is a machine and that is the problem. His muscles are so conditioned to handle the stress, they no longer need to adapt (or grow or get stronger). While training with him one day, we did his back routine, which entails five sets each of four different exercises with minimal rest between sets; however, I threw him a curve ball by insisting that we do the fourth exercise second and the second exercise fourth. Not surprisingly, Mike struggled like never before when he reached the third and fourth exercises. Something as simple as changing the exercise order delivered a different stimulus — it shocked his muscles thus leading to new adaptations.

To ensure maximum growth and symmetry, I change my training routine in some way almost every time I exercise. This is also important from a mental perspective, because changing your workouts can prevent stagnation. If you get bored with your routines, you will not bring maximum intensity and not stress the muscle enough to force an adaptation. In *Sports Supplement Review,* Bill Phillips recommends we rely on the following *principles of adaptation.*[5] After you learn the basic workouts provided in Chapters 11-14, I encourage you to create your own innovative workout plans and turn your training sessions into a process of self-discovery.

- *Choice of Exercise:* Using a variety of different exercises will allow you to hit specific muscles from all angles, leaving no area neglected.
- *Volume of Exercises*: When additional sets of the same exercise are added, muscle stimulation occurs through accumulation. By the fourth or fifth set fatigue causes the muscles to recruit fibers that you would otherwise not bring into play.
- *Super Sets*: With these sets the volume of intensity is raised by performing two different exercises that stress the same muscle group, one after the other.
- *Tri-sets*: The same theory applies as a third consecutive exercise is added that taxes one specific muscle group from different angles.

- *Number of Repetitions*: This will change in each of the program's six phases. Low reps will be used to hit the fast twitch fibers and high reps to tax the slow twitch fibers.
- *Rest between Exercises*: Such rest is also an important variable that will change, depending on objectives. Short rest periods provide endurance and fortify the body's ability to recover. Longer rest periods will be used during the bulking phase (5) because of the explosive, energy-sapping exercises you will be performing.
- *Tempo*: Each repetition is performed in three segments — the negative phase, where lowering one's body weight creates tension on the muscle; a pause, which is used to stretch the fascia or connective tissue; and the positive phase, where you contract and squeeze the muscle.
- *Change the Exercise Order*: Because you are stronger at the start of your workout, it is wise to begin with the heaviest resistance; however, starting a training session with the same exercise every time will plateau your progress, so you should change the order from time to time.
- *Rest between Workouts*: How many times you train during a given week is also an important variable that must be changed on a regular basis.

The Pump
When you perform high-intensity resistance training exercises, your muscles pump up like a balloon as a result of blood rushing into the muscle faster than your circulatory system can remove it. Blood is your body's primary system for transporting all the nutrients needed to support energy production, growth and recovery in muscle fibers. Blood is also responsible for removing lactic acid and carbon dioxide, metabolism byproducts that can inhibit performance and cause muscle fatigue. Thus, "the pump" is an important element for muscle development.

Neuromuscular Response
During the first four weeks of the *Hooked On Health* transformation program you will experience gains in strength before seeing visible signs of growth, since your body must first undergo a neuromuscular

response. With the body-weight resistance training exercises you create a stimulus within the central nervous system. This new activity is telegraphed from your brain to your muscles via the spinal cord and neurological pathways. Several workouts are required before your nervous system develops the neuro-motor communication necessary to recruit all the available muscle fibers.[6] For this reason, you should follow each exercise plan closely for four weeks before "mixing things up." Switching prematurely will prevent you from reaching your potential. But after four weeks, I encourage you to use any or even all of the principles of adaptation to keep your workouts fresh and challenging.

Hormonal Response
Hormones are chemical messengers produced by your endocrine system and released into the bloodstream. For muscle development and fat loss two categories of hormones are especially relevant: anabolic and catabolic. The anabolic hormones, testosterone, insulin, growth hormone and insulin-like growth factors (IGF-1) help build muscle proteins; the catabolic hormone, cortisol, helps break them down.[7] Following is a brief look at each of these hormones and the role they play in the muscle-development process. This information was adapted from Blair Whitmarsh's insightful book *Mind & Muscle*.

Testosterone is the most powerful anabolic hormone. Men have 10 times the amount of testosterone as women, and this is the primary reason that men develop greater muscle mass. Vigorous exercise, resistance training in particular, stimulates the production of testosterone. According to exercise physiologists, the largest surge in testosterone levels occur when (a) resistance is heavy – in the 3 to 7 repetition range, (b) rest intervals are short – 30 to 60 seconds, and (c) when you train the lower body. A lot of people (wrongly) assume that if they run, then they do not have to do resistance training for their legs. Hormones circulate throughout your entire body; therefore, working the legs, particularly with heavy squats, can lead to additional gains in muscle mass for your entire body.[8]

Insulin-like Growth Factors (IGF-1) play a less-understood role in muscle development, but increasing evidence indicates that the combined effects of growth hormone and IGF's are most responsible for the protein synthesis that leads to muscle growth. Growth hormone stimulates the production of IGF's in the cells of the muscle tissue, causing them to grow and possibly multiply (hyperplasia).[9]

Human Growth Hormone (HGH) functions include protein synthesis, fatty acid utilization, fat breakdown, glucose and amino acid release, and bone and cartilage growth.[10] Unfortunately, this wonder drug decreases as we age. HGH can be increased naturally through the same type of resistance training that is used to increase testosterone. It can also be increased through prescription human growth hormone (HGH) injections; however, Dr. Chopra advises against these injections due to numerous adverse effects. A number of nutritional supplements claim to cause the body to release HGH, but this claim is beyond the scope of my expertise. If you want to know more about these supplements and how they work, it is recommended that you read *Sports Supplement Review* by Bill Phillips.

Insulin is a carrier molecule that is released when you eat carbohydrate foods. When you digest a meal, the body converts protein into amino acids and carbohydrates into glucose, or blood sugar. Insulin then shuttles these nutrients into the muscles, where amino acids repair and develop new tissue; and glucose is converted into a stored form of energy called muscle glycogen. Thus, insulin helps your muscles and fat cells grow. *If muscle glycogen stores are full, insulin shuttles the nutrients into your fat cells.*[11] Therefore, it is critical that you to eat small meals. This important topic will be discussed it in greater detail in Chapter 6.

Cortisol, the so-called stress hormone, is catabolic and causes the body to break down muscle tissue and store body fat. Any kind of stress will trigger the release of cortisol: job-related anxiety, lack of food, worrying, lack of sleep and even exercise. With high-intensity resistance training the muscle fibers are "stressed" and go into a state of catabolism. Fortunately, exercise physiologists have discovered that consuming a post-workout meal containing both carbs and protein will shut down cortisol and immediately return the body to an anabolic, muscle-building state. Otherwise, it is important to eat regularly, get a good night's sleep and try to remove all stress from your life.[12]

Chapter

5

REST AND RECOVERY

For several days after an intense resistance-training workout your muscles will be inflamed and sore. In body-building circles this condition is commonly referred to as "delayed-onset muscle soreness" (DOMS) because you usually feel no pain until the next day. At this point rest is an essential component of muscle development. During the rest period your muscle fibers synthesize new proteins to repair the micro-tears and in doing so, they become bigger and stronger. This process takes at least 48 hours, sometimes longer. It is important to note that you should *never* train any muscle when it is sore, because (A) you can cause injury and (B) you will continue to tear down the muscle and short-circuit the development process. Muscles *only* grow during rest and recovery.

In a study conducted at Western Kentucky University (Bowling Green) scientists set out to discover exactly how long you should let a muscle recover before training it again. The findings, which were reported in *Muscle & Fitness* magazine by renowned science editors Jim Stoppani and Joe Wuebben, found that for many test subjects muscles fully recovered after just two days, but this isn't the case for everyone. By the third day, all of the participants had recovered, with many demonstrating increased strength. By the fourth day, most of the subjects displayed an increase in strength. The take home message: For most trainers, four days of recovery is optimal, yet some people may recover faster.[1]

Throughout the *Hooked On Health* training program, workouts are split, so that we train one group of muscles while another group rests and recovers. For example, during Phase 2 our resistance training split will be: Monday — chest, shoulders and triceps; Wednesday — legs; Friday — back, biceps, abs. Training splits turn up the metabolic furnace, because at least one body part is constantly repairing itself and burning fat in the process.

The significance of the rest and recovery phase is exemplified by the training philosophy of Athletes' Performance Institute, a state-of-the-art-athletic training facility located on the campus of Arizona State University. The Institute, frequented by numerous professional athletes, teaches its high-profile clients that recovery is the limiting factor in performance. In fact, half of the building is called work and the other half is called rest. To ensure optimal muscle regeneration, the facility provides steam rooms, heat treatment, hydrotherapy, electronic muscle stimulation and an array of massage therapy techniques. If America's best trainers and athletes consider rest to be as important as the workout, then you should too.

Sleep is arguably the most important factor in recovery, because during sleep is when most of the cellular changes and growth occur. According to a study published by researchers at Columbia University,[2] sleep is also a critical factor in weight loss. The 6,000-person study revealed that obesity rates were 23 percent greater in people who slept an average of six hours a night (as opposed to the seven to eight hours logged by regular sleepers); and a dramatic 73 percent higher in people who slept only two to four hours a night.

In an article that appeared in *Men's Health* magazine titled "Good Luck and Good Night" columnist Peter Moore explains how a lack of sleep causes people to gain weight: "Researchers at the University of Chicago have been tracking the correlation between sleep and two hunger hormones: ghrelin, which urges your body to chow down; and leptin, which tells it to push back from the table. They recruited 12 young men and limited them to four hours of sleep on two consecutive nights. It was as if they'd cut their hunger brake lines and attached a brick on the accelerators: ghrelin was up 28 percent and leptin was down 18 percent."[3]

According to scientists at the National Sleep Foundation, a 20-minute power nap increases mental acuity and muscle responsiveness. I take a 10-20 minute nap immediately after my post-workout meal and have found this to be true. Short naps shut down cortisol and allow the body to focus on repairing the micro-tears in muscle fibers. If you do nap, try not to exceed 20 minutes, because long naps can disrupt your nighttime sleep.

The Athletes' Performance Institute highly recommends massage to reduce soreness and help muscles recover faster. I actually give myself a 10-minute massage every morning and it definitely helps. Massage may also promote muscle growth, because it encourages the body to release human growth hormone. In a fascinating experiment Dr. Tiffany Fields of the Touch Research Institute at the University of Miami School of Medicine found that preemie babies who were given a daily massage gained 47 percent more weight than preemies who did not receive massage therapy during the first six weeks after birth. Other benefits of massage include increased circulation, lower blood pressure and relaxed muscles.[4] Plan to make massage therapy part of your new lifestyle. If you can afford the costs, get a massage at least once a week. If your finances do not allow for weekly trips to a therapist, buy a good "How to Massage" video and offer to trade off with a friend or family member. Or you can do it yourself.

Another excellent way to reduce soreness and speed up recovery is to stretch every day. Stretching brings freshly oxygenated blood, vitamins, minerals and other nutrients to inflamed muscle fibers and elongates muscles, reduces lactic acid buildup and strengthens connective joint tissue.[5]

Sore muscles also respond well to heat. Sitting in a Jacuzzi, sauna, steam room or warm bath will soothe these aching muscles. Saunas and steam treatments are also an important weight loss aid, because fat tissues release stored toxins.[6] These toxins lower your T3 levels, consequently slowing your resting metabolic rate and inhibiting your fat burning ability.[7]

6

PROPER NUTRITION

Proper nutrition is equally as important as a high-intensity exercise program if you want to lose weight and develop a lean, muscular physique. This part of the *Hooked On Health* formula is also based on medical science's latest discoveries and is critical to achieving your fitness objectives.

In order to clearly understand the role diet plays in weight loss and muscle development, we begin with a recap of how metabolism works. During digestion, enzymes split proteins into amino acids, which are the building blocks of new cell tissues, and carbohydrates into glucose (blood sugar). At this time the body releases a hormone called insulin, whose job is to transport these compounds to the cells via the bloodstream.[1] Once it reaches the cells, amino acids repair or replace tissues; glucose can be converted into a stored form of energy called glycogen, or it can enter the mitochondria where it will be turned into energy. If you eat too much in one sitting, all of the excess calories will be stored in adipose tissues — the body's back-up energy supply.

Fat loss occurs when you achieve a negative energy balance. Decreasing the total number of calories you consume and increasing your energy expenditure normally accomplish this loss. The goal of proper nutrition is to achieve a negative energy balance, and burn fat for fuel, without allowing the body to burn muscle. In order to accomplish this objective, it is imperative that you eat small, frequent meals (every two to three hours). Researchers have demonstrated through numerous studies that athletes who eat three times a day have significantly higher levels of body fat compared to those who eat six times a day. The reason for these levels is that frequent meals even out blood sugar, preventing peaks and valleys that cause your body to defend fat stores.[2] When you eat large meals, your body cannot absorb all the nutrients, and therefore uses what it needs and "stores" the rest as fat for times of famine.

One of the leading researchers on weight loss and nutrient timing is Jeff Volek, PhD, the author of the book *TNT Diet* and a professor at the University of Connecticut. In an article that appeared in *Men's Health* magazine he explains why small, frequent meals— and a low carb diet—are so important for weight loss:

> **Your glycogen tank has a limited capacity to store carbs. Think of your car: If it's a midsize, it probably has a 14-gallon fuel tank. Try to fill the tank with 20 gallons, and the extra six will spill out onto the pavement. It's the same way with carbs and your glycogen tank.**
>
> **So this is where the problem lies: Once your glycogen tank is full, the excess carbs you eat overflow into your bloodstream and are shuttled off to your liver, where they're converted into fat.[3]**

When you eat in relation to your workouts is also an integral part of the muscle development and fat loss equation. You cannot exercise vigorously on an empty tank, so about one or two hours before exercising, you should eat a meal in order to fill your energy (glycogen) stores. Research shows that consuming a *low-fat* pre-workout meal consisting of both protein and carbohydrates reduces the stress response that occurs when muscle fibers are torn. According to a University of Maryland School of Medicine study, a *high-fat* meal will blunt the ability of nitric oxide, another body chemical, to open blood vessels for up to four hours.[4] This reaction is critical, because proper blood flow — the pump — is important for muscle growth. A high fat meal will also cause a 50 percent reduction in post-workout growth hormone release. Growth hormone is important for both muscle development and fat burning. Thus, the pre-workout meal must be low in fat.

In Chapter 4 we learned that high-intensity resistance training is a "stress" that causes the body to release the hormone, cortisol. A high level of cortisol inhibits glucose from getting into cells, causing the muscles to break down. Therefore, it is imperative that you immediately shut down cortisol by consuming a post-workout protein shake and a high-glycemic carbohydrate. The glycemic index is discussed below. This type of carb will "spike" insulin, which shuts down cortisol and also replenishes glycogen stores, enabling all of the protein to be synthesized for muscle growth.[5]

From a muscle development perspective, the two meals following your workout are by far the most important. There is a short window of opportunity immediately after the workout when nutrients are rapidly and efficiently absorbed by muscle fibers. Therefore, to achieve optimal results, you need to eat something as soon as you complete your training session. With this meal you will want a fast-digesting source of protein. A protein shake is best, but if you must go with whole food, choose egg whites or tuna. The carb source needs to be from the high-glycemic category, which will release more insulin from your pancreas to ensure optimal nutrient uptake. About an hour or two later eat a balanced meal with lots of protein (fish, turkey, or chicken), sufficient healthy carbs (wild rice, whole-wheat pasta) and a fibrous green vegetable.

After cardio workouts you should wait an hour before eating. This waiting forces your body — which has depleted its glycogen stores — to burn fat for fuel. If you choose to wait an hour before eating after a cardio workout, you must be aware that there is a fine line between burning fat and breaking down muscle tissue for energy. The body will tap the fat stores first; however, if activity is too high it may also begin to cannibalize muscle.

It is also advisable to reduce carbs after dinner. Late-night carbs are twice as likely to be converted into fat because activity levels decrease significantly after dinner. The only exception would be if you did your resistance training workouts in the evening; in this case you *must* consume your post-workout carbs. In fact, if you are one of those people who is unwilling to give up their evening couch potato munchies, you should consider evening workouts. Although not the best time to exercise and consume nutrients, the workout will reduce the negative effects of late-night carbs.

Protein

For optimal results, Bill Phillips recommends a high protein diet consisting of 40 percent protein, 40 percent carbohydrates, and 20 percent fat. He suggests that people eat six meals daily consisting of one fist-size portion of protein and one fist-size portion of carbs.[6] A significantly large body of science now exists to support the effectiveness of Phillips' meal plan for muscle development and fat loss. For example, a study published in a 2006 issue of *Muscle & Fitness* found that test subjects who got 40 percent of total daily calories from protein, while also following a weight training and cardio program, lost more than twice as much body fat as those getting just 15-20 percent of total daily calories from protein and following a cardio-only exercise program.[7]

The goal of the Hooked On Health system is to help you lose body fat while simultaneously gaining lean muscle. This is made possible through appropriate training and calorie restriction.[8] Rapid weight loss following calorie restriction can result in losses of lean body mass. To counteract the potential for muscular losses and a subsequent decrease in metabolic rate during calorie restriction, resistance training and an increase in dietary protein should accompany attempts at weight loss.[9]

To figure out how much protein you should consume, simply multiply .08 times your body weight. I weigh 200 pounds so my daily requirement is 160 grams of protein. Divide this requirement by six meals and you get approximately 25 grams per meal. I usually try to get about 35 grams of protein in each of my two post-workout meals. Otherwise, most of my meals are in the 20 to 30-gram range. Most bodybuilder magazines recommend 1 to 1.5 grams of protein per pound of body weight for optimal muscle development. On a prison diet, I do not have access to that much protein, and personally I do not want enormous muscles, but if you do, then I suggest you follow the bodybuilder guidelines. Bottom line: Protein is made up of 20 amino acids, and the aminos are what develop muscle tissue.

According to some researchers, the source of the protein you consume will have dramatic effects on your long-term health. One such expert is T. Colin Campbell, Ph.D., the author of *The China Study*, a book considered to be the most comprehensive study on nutrition ever conducted. Campbell, who is Professor Emeritus of Nutritional Biochemistry at Cornell University, the author of 350 scientific articles, and the recipient of the 1998 American Institute of Cancer Research award "in recognition of a lifetime of significant accomplishments in scientific research," has conducted experimental animal studies, funded by grants from the National Institutes of Health, for more than four decades. In one landmark study, Campbell demonstrated unequivocally that casein protein (derived from cow's milk) caused cancer in rats. He writes:

> Rats generally live for about two years, thus the study was 100 weeks in length. All animals that were administered aflatoxin (a cancer-causing agent) and fed the 20% casein diet were either dead or near death from liver tumors at 100 weeks. All animals administered the same level of aflatoxin but fed the low 5% casein protein diet were alive, active and thrifty, with sleek hair coats at 100 weeks. This was a virtual 100 to 0 score, something almost never seen in research... Soy protein and gluten, the protein of wheat, did not produce the same toxic result as casein, even when fed at the same 20% level.[10]

Campbell's research demonstrated that protein derived from cows is a primary cause of cancer and heart disease. Several other prominent health researchers, including Dr. Dean Ornish, Dr. William Castelli, and Dr. Caldwell Esselstyn, concur. In the fantastic book *Ultra Prevention,* Dr. Mark Hyman and Dr. Mark Liponis advise against consuming milk or red meat because "American" beef cattle are contaminated with antibiotics, hormones, and unnatural food sources designed to fatten them up. Interestingly, they write: "Argentina's range-fed beef cattle eat wild plants, so the content of saturated fat in their tissues is 500% less than grain-fed beef cattle. Saturated fats lead to fatty buildup in the walls of your arteries."[11] Cows were not meant to be injected with hormones and antibiotics, or eat grains. The results have been disastrous to our health.

Acclaimed novelist Jonathon Safron Foer weighed in on the subject in the new book *Eating Animals.* In an interview with *USA Today's* Elizabeth Weise, he says:

> My book is not a case for vegetarianism. It's a case against factory farmed meat. Basically, that's meat where animals are raised in enclosures, where they don't get to see the sun, don't get to touch the Earth, and they're almost always fed drugs to keep them from getting sick or make them grow faster.[12]

Foer talks about the sheer misery of cows and chickens being confined to cages so small that they cannot even turn around. As a man who is incarcerated and has been confined to small cages, I can attest to the misery and the resulting stress. There is no doubt in my mind that these conditions cause the animals to secrete stress hormones which also have toxic effects on the meat (as well as milk and eggs) that we find at the supermarket.

What's a meat-loving American supposed to do to meet his body's protein requirements? In *The Perricone Weight Loss Diet,* Dr. Nicholas Perricone suggests:

> **If you want to eat meat, follow these safety guidelines. First, try to buy only organic meat raised from animals that are free of antibiotics and hormones, whose feed is free of potentially dangerous chemicals — ideally animals (including poultry) will be free-range — that is, not raised in feed lots, but out in a pasture.**[13]

Not all protein sources have been contaminated by the practices of the farmed meat industry. Lean meats, including deer, bison, ostrich, gator, elk, buffalo, and all kinds of seafood are excellent sources or protein. Significant quantities of protein may also be found in many plant foods, including beans, lentils, tofu, soy, and wheat. Most bodybuilders will be surprised to learn that there are 12 grams of protein in 100 calories of spinach compared to 13 grams of protein in a porterhouse steak.[14] You do not have to be a carnivore or risk your long-term health to get the quantity of protein required to develop large muscles.

Carbohydrates

When it comes to developing your best body and achieving optimal health, carbohydrates are just as important as protein. In fact, if you do not maintain a steady flow of carbs, your energy level will plummet and you will lose muscle mass. As noted above, carbohydrates are converted into muscle glycogen, the body's primary energy source. When glycogen levels drop, exercise capacity is impaired; this in turn prevents you from training at the intensity levels necessary for muscle development and fat loss. Worse yet, when energy stores are empty, the body first tries to burn fat; however, if the fat burning is too slow to provide the necessary energy, your body will become catabolic and begin to break down muscles for fuel.

The carbohydrates you want to avoid are those found in processed foods, such as white bread, white rice, white pasta, sugary cereals, cookies, chips, cakes, crackers, candy, and other snack foods.

The consumption of refined carbohydrates found in processed foods is the primary reason that so many Americans are overweight. These man-made junk foods wreak havoc on the metabolism.

Refined carbohydrates are high-glycemic. The glycemic index (GI) is a numerical scale that describes how fast a carbohydrate food is metabolized into blood sugar. Man-made junk foods are digested far too quickly, flooding your system with more blood sugar than it can process. The other problem with refined carbs is that they "spike" your insulin secretion. When insulin is over-secreted too frequently, the body becomes insulin resistant. For more insight into this phenomenon, consider the following passage from *Dr. Atkins New Diet Revolution:*

> **What appears to happen is the insulin receptors on the surfaces of the body's cells are blocked, which in turn prevents glucose from reaching the cells for energy use. That's one reason why overweight individuals may be tired much of the time. When insulin is ineffective at taking glucose into the cells, the liver converts more and more glucose into stored body fat. Your body is, in fact, becoming a fat producing machine instead of an efficient energy producing machine.**
>
> **Your body's hormonal system is now in desperate straits. At this point, insulin is being secreted more and more frequently to deal with high blood sugar levels, and it is doing its job less and less effectively. Which makes you crave sweets and carbs, which compounds the problem in a vicious cycle. In time, even the insulin receptors that convert glucose to fat start getting worn out, forecasting diabetes.[15]**

"Refined carbs are the primary cause of Type II diabetes!" So said British Surgeon Captain T.L. Cleve, MD. In the book, *Saccharine Disease: The Master Disease of Our Time,* Cleve examined nearly a dozen cultures in which diabetes simply never occurred until 20 years after people in that culture began to consume significant amounts of refined carbohydrates.[16]

Cleve also argues that increases in the incidents of heart disease can be traced directly to increased consumption of refined carbohydrates.[17] This insight is supported by the Harvard Nurses Study, the largest, long-term epidemiological study being conducted in America.

The Harvard researchers, led by Walter Willett, tracked the dietary and health habits of more than 10,000 nurses for two decades. Their findings: eating foods high on the glycemic index leads to elevated blood sugar and insulin levels, which in turn leads to hypertension, undesirable cholesterol and triglyceride levels, and other risk factors associated with heart disease.[18]

In a *Men's Health* special report titled "The Cure for Diabetes" columnist Adam Campbell writes: "Diabetes is the primary cause of cardiovascular disease, slashing a man's lifespan by an average of 13 years." Campbell's report describes the work of Dr. Mary Vernon, a family doctor who has successfully helped more than 50 patients reverse diabetes simply by changing their eating habits. Dr. Vernon says: "I believe in addressing the cause, not the symptoms. That's why I eliminate the foods that raise blood sugar. It's only logical." Researchers at Duke University set out to test Dr. Vernon's findings in a laboratory setting. The results of their 16-week study were striking: 17 out of 21 diabetic patients who participated in the study were able to significantly reduce their medication or discontinue it altogether.[19]

I shared these insights with a woman named Lety who had recently been diagnosed with diabetes and was 30 pounds overweight. I told Lety that I thought she might be able to overcome her diabetes by following the diet and exercise recommendations in the book I was writing titled *Penitentiary Fitness*. (Other research indicates that mitochondrial damage caused by eating processed junk foods contributes to diabetes, and that high-intensity exercises can sometimes restore the mitochondria to normal function.) Lety embraced the idea enthusiastically and even agreed to complete before and after physicals to document the results. I mailed Lety a copy of the manuscript and just 90 days after beginning the program she had completely reversed the disease. She was able to stop taking both her diabetes medication and her blood pressure medication, and she lost 22 pounds of body fat. Her before and after blood test results were remarkable. All of the diabetes biomarkers dropped significantly: glucose from 235 to 128; AST from 130 to 81; and ALT from 147 to 91. Moreover, the two most significant benchmarks for heart disease also fell into the normal range: total cholesterol from 242 to 198; and triglycerides from 132 to 108.

The carbohydrates that you want to eat are those found in nature. All plant-based foods are rich in phytonutrients, which are essential for achieving optimal health. These phytonutrients turn the genes that control weight and metabolism on and off, and help prevent every known chronic disease of modern civilization.[20] Most plant-based foods are also high in fiber, which slows the entry of glucose into the bloodstream. This in turn reduces the blood sugar spikes that cause insulin production and encourage the body to produce and store body fat.[21] Healthy plant-based foods include nuts, seeds, whole grains, vegetables and fruits.

Nuts and seeds are tasty, healthy food sources excellent for muscle development and weight loss. In addition to being a healthy source of carbs, they are rich in protein and good fats that promote satiety. They are also rich in nutrients that minimize your risk of heart disease. One study, published in the *British Medical Journal,* found that eating a minimum of five ounces of nuts and seeds per week reduced heart attacks by 33 percent.[22]

Whole grain foods also play a role in the quest for optimal health. They increase the movement of food through the digestive system, lower cholesterol levels, and are an important source of antioxidants. Whole grain foods include bread, tortillas, pasta, rice, English muffins, bagels, oatmeal and some cold cereals. It is important to know which brands to buy and this topic will be discussed in Chapter 7.

Vegetables also play an important role in maintaining proper nutrition. Green vegetables in particular will help your body fight heart disease and cancer and also neutralize free radicals — molecules that accelerate the aging process. Spinach and broccoli have the highest concentration of antioxidants, but really all vegetables are densely packed with vitamins and minerals. For individuals looking to lose weight, there is nothing, and I repeat, nothing better than loading your plate with veggies such as asparagus, broccoli, Brussels sprouts, spinach, cabbage, collards, cauliflower, green beans, squash and zucchini. The reason that vegetables are so good for weight loss is because they are low in calories.

Fruit is also low in calories and a good food choice for people who want to shed body fat. It is excellent as the only carb source in a small meal. At least one of my meals every day consists of one piece of fruit and a protein shake. With this meal I usually try to eat Select Fruits (a term we will be using later) — oranges, apples, grapefruit, peaches and berries. These select fruits contain pectin, a soluble fiber that expands in the stomach and makes you feel full longer.

The glycemic index is an excellent tool for people who are looking to lose weight; however, it is not perfect. The anomalies to the system are the Healthy High Glycemics, foods such as baked potatoes, watermelon, and tropical fruits, which are low in calories and good for you. These are the high GI carbs that are recommended for the post resistance training workout meal. Post-workout is the *only* time it's actually good to spike your insulin and blood sugar levels because muscles will be inflamed and screaming for nutrients. Healthy High Glycemics shut down post-workout cortisol levels and replenish muscle glycogen stores.

If you want to be healthy and live a long life, then you need to eat lots of whole grains, nuts, seeds, fruits and vegetables. Plant-based foods are loaded with vitamins, minerals, fiber and disease-fighting phyto-nutrients. Plant-based foods are also one of the best you can eat to fight heart disease, because they contain bioflavonoids, which prevent the blood from thickening and clogging the arteries. Some people assume that because they take vitamins, they do not necessarily need to eat a lot of whole grains, fruits and vegetables, but this is untrue because vitamins do not contain bioflavonoids or phytonutrients.

Following is a general listing of both healthy and unhealthy carbohydrate foods:

CARBS

Healthy Carbs	Unhealthy Carbs
Plums/apples/cherries/pineapple	Fruit juice (not freshly squeezed)
Grapefruit/grapes/kiwi	White bread/French fries
Oranges/peaches/pears/mango	White rice/pretzels
Strawberries/bananas	Bagels/macaroni and cheese
All types of melon	Corn flakes/corn chips
Lentils/whole corn	Croissants
Beans/peas	Cake
Potatoes with skin/popcorn	Candy
Oatmeal/brown or wild rice	Sugary drinks
Whole wheat pasta/fat-free milk	Beer
Bran cereal/barley	Instant flavored oatmeal

Fats

The final piece to the dietary puzzle is fat. And like carbs, there are good fats and bad fats. One specific type of fat, omega-3 fatty acids, is particularly important for maintaining cardiovascular health. In an Italian study of 11,323 heart attack survivors, researchers found that those taking a daily fish oil capsule containing omega-3 fatty acids were 42 percent less likely to suffer a second heart attack than those not taking the supplement.[23] In the *Perricone Weight Loss Diet* Dr. Nicholas Perricone describes the significant health benefits of omega-3 fatty acids: stabilize blood sugar levels, lower insulin levels, increase immunological function, improve attention span, elevate mood, increase radiance of skin, increase energy levels, and decrease symptoms and severity of rheumatoid arthritis.[24]

Some fats are also important for weight loss. Most people are unaware of this fact because food manufacturers' marketing of low-fat products has created a belief that the fats in foods lead to excess fat on our bodies. In fact, the opposite is true with certain types of fat. Consider the following insights from Dr. Hyman's wonderful book, *Ultra Metabolism:*

> **Some key fats (omega-3) enter the cells and communicate with your DNA to turn on special genes that help you increase fat burning, improve your blood sugar control, correct insulin, and reduce inflammation.[25]**

After learning these scientific facts about the omega-3 fats found in fish, I began to wonder what would happen if a person made fish the centerpiece of their diet. The combination of Dr. Hyman's research and my curiosity inspired a unique weight loss experiment. First, I gorged myself for two months, gaining 25 pounds of body fat. Next, I challenged two of the fittest guys on the prison yard to a six-week "Best Abs" contest. I was so overweight that you couldn't even see my abs, so they leaped at the opportunity to take my money. During the six-week contest, I ate mackerel four times a day. Two of these meals were a piece of fish and a piece of fruit. Following insights from Dr. Volek's *TNT Diet,* my two snacks were just a piece of fish because "limiting carbohydrate consumption trains the body to use fat as its primary source of energy."[26] For the other two meals, breakfast and dinner, I ate whatever healthy food that was available at the chow hall.

The results were truly extraordinary. Not only did I lose all of the unwanted body fat, but I also achieved a lean, muscular physique beyond my wildest aspirations. Moreover, this transformation occurred at the age of 42, when the metabolism is supposed to be slowing down. Have you ever wondered why participants on the TV program "Survivor" lose so much body fat? It's because the lean combination of fish and fruit is a magical weight loss elixir and because they have no access to processed junk foods.

The Omega-3 Fish Diet described above was also inexpensive. From the prison canteen I purchased a large can of mackerel, containing 78 grams of lean protein for one dollar. Of course, there are tastier types of fish that are high in omega-3 fatty acids, including salmon, black cod (aka sablefish), trout, herring, sardines, and tuna. If you don't like eating fish, you can get the omega-3's from fish oil supplements, flaxseeds, or walnuts. There is even an omega-3-packed dessert topping called Coromega that can be mixed with yogurt.

The other healthy fats are the monounsaturated and poly-unsaturated fats found in plant foods. Olive oil is particularly rich in antioxidants. These healthy fats play a key role in satiety and the distribution of soluble vitamins. The fats to avoid are saturated fats and trans fats. Following is a partial list from each category:

FATS

Unsaturated Fats	Saturated Fats	Trans Fats
Fish	Whole milk	Any fried foods
Nuts	Cheese	Margarine/cheese spread
Avocados	Butter	Candy bars
Soybeans	Cream	Cookies
Olive oil	Red meat	Potato chips

Saturated fats, mostly found in red meat, butter, and full-fat dairy products, promote heart disease and cancer. Saturated fat leads to the buildup of plaque in the walls of the arteries. Plaque is a foreign substance that collects in the arteries and can lead to heart disease later in life.

Trans fats are even worse, acting like a time-released poison that is slowly killing you. Trans fat is a man-made substance. Since this substance is not found in nature, our system does not recognize it or process it very well.

Scientists at Harvard University conducted an 80,000-person study that was designed to investigate the harmful effects of trans fat. Check out what they found.[27] Trans fats:

- May contribute to as many as 30,000 premature deaths each year.
- Dramatically increase the amount of bad cholesterol in the blood.
- Lower HDL (good) cholesterol.
- Weaken your immune system.
- Can cause the risk of heart disease to go up 50 percent if more than three percent of the daily calories come from trans fat.
- People with the highest daily intake of trans fat have the highest incidence of diabetes.

Shortly after these findings were published, the Institute of Medicine advised that all Americans should reduce their consumption of foods made with hydrogenated oils. The best way to tell if a food has trans fat is by searching the ingredients list for "partially hydrogenated oils." To help you avoid these rancid fats, following is a listing for foods that contain a lot of trans fat:

TRANS-FAT FOODS

Packaged cookies /candy
Packaged doughnuts, pies, cakes
Non-dairy creamers/whipped toppings
Most dry cereal (not whole grain)
Certain types of protein/energy bars
Fried foods, chips, crackers
Margarine, dried soups, frozen dinners

Snacks and Maintaining Satiety

As mentioned at the beginning of Chapter 6, you should consume a meal every two to three hours to maintain a steady supply of energy and balance your insulin secretion. Ideally, you should have a healthy meal containing protein and carbohydrates for breakfast, lunch and dinner. You will also want to have a mid-morning and mid-afternoon snack to prevent you from becoming ravenously hungry and overeating. If you keep portion sizes small, you can even have a late-evening snack.

When I initially started eating small, frequent meals, I encountered a problem with satiety — feeling unsatisfied and hungry immediately after eating. I later learned that I felt this way because my stomach was stretched from eating larger meals. The stomach has an elastic quality to it, so if you are used to eating larger meals, you will not get full from a small meal. However, once you train yourself to eat small meals, the stomach will actually shrink and adjust to the new eating pattern, normally in a couple of weeks. Also, as the stomach fills up, the body produces a hormone called ghrelin which sends a "full" signal to the brain in a period of up to 20 minutes. This slow signal is one of the reasons that a lot of us overeat. You can minimize the hunger pangs frequently experienced during this 20-minute window by taking smaller bites, chewing food longer, savoring tastes and frequently sipping water.

The healthiest food sources for the mid-morning, mid-afternoon, and evening snacks are nuts and fruits. Nuts are the perfect unit of food since they contain protein, carbs, and healthy fats. Fruit is low in calories and high in fiber. Perhaps the healthiest snack of all are berries (strawberries, blueberries, raspberries, cranberries, blackberries). Berries contain the highest anti-oxidant profile of any food source. At only 50 calories for a one-cup serving, they are the ideal snack for anyone trying to lose weight.

The Importance of Breakfast

Over the last 20 years the field of "crono-biology" has studied the effect of the 24-hour cycle on the human body, known as circadian rhythms. This study reveals how human life functions in relation to time. Crono-biologists have discovered that breakfast "sets" your metabolism for the remainder of the day.

Researchers at the University of Texas analyzed the effect of circadian rhythms on food consumption, and found that eating more calories earlier in the day reduces overall food intake. The researchers also learned that foods with a higher nutrient density (those found in nature) are more satiating.[28]

Another fascinating breakfast study, conducted by Harvard professor Dr. David Ludwig, compared the effects of meal composition. One group ate instant oatmeal; the second group ate steel cut oats (not instant); the third group ate a vegetable omelet and a piece of fruit. Even though each breakfast meal contained the same number of calories, the instant oatmeal group felt hungrier and consumed 81 percent more calories later that day than was consumed by the vegetable omelet and fruit group. The steel cut oats group consumed 51 percent more calories than the vegetable omelet group. Their blood tests tell the whole story: the instant oatmeal group had the highest levels of insulin and blood sugar; the steel cut oats group was the second highest, and the vegetable omelet group was by far the lowest.[29]

The wisdom distilled from these two studies is that eating a healthy, balanced, nutrient-rich breakfast is crucial for weight loss. Remember, how well your metabolism functions is directly related to how effectively your insulin transports blood sugar to the mitochondria for energy production. Even a healthy food source such as oatmeal will disrupt your metabolism when it is processed to become an "instant food." When you eat plant-based carbs and lean protein together, blood sugar and insulin stabilize, enabling your metabolism to function at peak efficiency.

Hydration = cell volumization = muscle growth
Water is the most important nutrient in the quest for optimal health. Without adequate water intake, the cardiovascular system will not function properly. In their informative book *Sports Supplements,* J. Stout and J. Antonio explain:

> **Blood serves to transport nutrients to every cell in the human body. Hydrostatic pressure is the primary force that propels blood through the arteries, thus controlling cardiac output. Adequate blood volume is one requirement for maintaining hydrostatic pressure and adequate body water is needed to maintain blood volume; thus, the amount of body water has a direct effect on hydrostatic pressure. In addition, muscular metabolism, hormonal responses, and kidney function may also be affected by dehydration.[30]**

According to a study published in the journal *Obesity Research,* guys who drink the most water each day take in an average of 194 fewer calories a day than guys who drink less water. Over the course of a year, those savings could help you drop up to 20 pounds.[31]

A glass of water contains zero calories.

Exchanging soda, coffee, alcohol, and iced tea for water causes something amazing to happen within the body. With the exception of a cup of green tea in the morning and another before workouts, the *only* beverage you should drink is water. Following this advice can make all the difference in how you feel and look.

Proper hydration also plays a major role in the process of muscle development. It is important to drink water before, during and after workouts because intense exercise depletes the amount of hydrating nutrients in the muscle cells. Drinking a full liter of water during the 90 minutes before your workout is ideal. Also hit the water fountain after every five sets. If it's a humid day and you are sweating a lot, drink after every two sets.

It is a good rule to drink two 12-ounce glasses of water with every meal. If you follow this simple guideline your body will be hyper-hydrated and I guarantee you will feel positive changes in your health within a week.

Chapter

7

THE CONNECT WITH NATURE WEIGHT LOSS SOLUTION

"Necessity is the mother of all invention." For me, this timeless maxim has become a profound truth because it was through necessity that I discovered the ultimate fat-burning diet solution. As mentioned earlier, hip and low back injuries prevent me from doing any high-intensity interval training aerobic activities, thus I was having difficulty shedding my love handles. Then the prison decided to do construction on the building where I was "housed," and I was forced to remain outside on the prison yard from 8:00 a.m. until 4:00 p.m. every day for two weeks.

Normally I spend most of my day researching and writing, tasks that do not require a large expenditure of energy. But during that two-week period outdoors, I took a lot of long walks. The end result was that I burned more calories than I consumed, and that caused my body to tap its fat stores to fuel the extra activity. The love handles completely disappeared.

Shortly thereafter I read an interesting weight loss study[1] in which participants were instructed to walk 10,000 steps a day (roughly five miles) without changing their diets. The researchers used a pedometer, a device that counts the number of steps taken. After six months test subjects lost an average of 24 pounds, which is approximately one pound per week.

One pound of body fat is equal to 3,500 calories, therefore, the study's test subjects were burning about 500 calories per day above their body's energy needs as a result of walking 10,000 steps. I quickly surmised that they could have doubled their weight loss by also reducing their calorie intake by 500 calories per day. It became clear to me that optimal weight loss would occur when a person works both sides of the energy balance equation. Burn more energy by increasing activity levels and consume less energy by making smart food choices.

This revelation inspired me to create a simple, two-part weight loss solution. The first part of the weight loss solution is to burn 500 calories a day (above and beyond exercise and regular activities) through short, well-planned walks. Purchase a pedometer and work your way up to 10,000 steps daily. For those working a typical nine-to-five job, I recommend that you optimize your break periods. Many employers offer a lunch hour and a 15-minute mid-morning and mid-afternoon break. Use the majority of this time to go outdoors, connect with nature, and walk. The combination of fresh air, sunshine, and physical activity will be much more energizing than lounging around. If you prepare your meals ahead of time, it will not take long to eat them. You could easily get 30-40 minutes of walking in during the lunch hour and another 10 at each of your breaks.

If you work in an office building, you can increase your calorie burn by walking the stairs. Fill a backpack with books, put it on, and you can crank the burn up even higher. Increase your energy expenditure by taking on some hills or adding squat, lunge, or jumping jack intervals every minute or two.

Chapter 7's title, "The Connect With Nature Weight Loss Solution," was chosen because the key to fat burning and optimal health lies in the complete elimination of man-made processed foods. In addition to disrupting body chemistry and creating disease, processed foods are loaded with extra calories that have absolutely no nutritional value. For example, a five-strip order of McDonald's Chicken Select Premium Breast Strips has 630 calories – a 3-oz. serving of salmon has 80; two Mrs. Fields Milk Chocolate & Walnuts cookies have 650 calories – a huge bowl of fresh strawberries about 100; a Pepperidge Farms Chicken Pot Pie has 1,010 calories – a salad with strips of chicken without the skin, maybe 350; and a large order of Burger King French fries has 600 calories – a large bowl of asparagus spears less than 100. The calorie comparison between processed foods and foods found in nature is fairly dramatic. Moreover, processed foods are chock-full of artery-clogging fats that create heart disease, and foods found in nature are rich in antioxidants that fight disease.

Another consideration is that human beings are part of the circle of life. Consider the following insights from Dr. Deepak Chopra's audio series *Training the Mind — Healing the Body:*

> In the course of one year, 99 percent of the atoms that make up your body are *exchanged* with the environment. New cell tissues are formed from foods that come from Mother Earth. We eat animal, vegetable or mineral products and organize them into more complex structures that make up our bones, organs, tissues and skin. When we die, all goes back to the earth.[2]

The problem that arises with processed food is that its molecular structure has been altered, and our systems do not recognize it. When you eat a cookie your body says, "What the heck is this? I can't make a new liver or tooth out of this, but just in case there is a famine, I'll store it over here (fat cells) in my backup energy supply."

The second part of this weight loss solution involves selecting the most energy efficient foods, which are those found in nature. The source of our food's energy is the sun. Through a complex process called "photosynthesis" living plants take the energy of the sun and transform it into life.[3] We get our energy either by consuming the plants directly or by consuming the animals that feed on the plants. Provided the animals are not factory farmed — meaning that they were raised by farmers outside in a natural environment — both plants and animals are good sources of energy for humans. Yet some leading weight loss researchers argue that plant-based foods are more energy efficient. These arguments have merit on two accounts.

The first is energy density. In *The Perricone Weight Loss Diet*, Dr. Nicholas Perricone explains:

> Eating foods with a low energy density can support a healthy body weight because they make you feel satisfied with fewer calories. Energy density is the amount of calories in a portion of food. Because of their high water and fiber content, avocados (and other plant foods) are considered a low energy density food — few calories per ounce. By filling up on foods with a low energy density, satiety is achieved with fewer calories.[4]

The other reason plant based foods are considered to be optimal for energy efficiency is their ability to encourage physical activity. T. Colin Campbell's research on animals whose diets consisted of low, five percent or high 20 percent casein (animal protein) proves to be informative. In *The China Study* he writes:

Some of us had noticed over the course of these experiments that the 5% casein animals seemed to be more active than the 20% animals. To test this idea, we housed rats fed either 5% or 20% casein diets in cages equipped with exercise wheels outfitted with meters to record the number of turns of the wheel. *Within the very first day the 5% casein-fed animals voluntarily "exercised" in the wheel about twice as much as the 20% casein-fed animals.* Exercise remained considerably higher for the 5% casein animals throughout the two weeks of the study.[5]

The research clearly indicates that plant based foods should be a significant part of your diet if your goal is to lose weight. You can also mix in some lean, free-range animal based proteins. The foods you want to avoid are the processed foods and the factory farmed animal products. If you are someone who enjoys animal foods such as beef, poultry, eggs, and dairy products, then I highly recommend that you purchase these foods at farmer's markets. My one guiding principle on food is this: If God made it; if it can be found within the circle of life; it's good for you. But if man has created the food through industrial processing or has tampered with it in any way, it's probably not good for you.

The primary objective in creating the Connect With Nature Weight Loss Solution was to create a healthy nutrition plan that would keep transformation aspirants in a muscle-building, fat-burning state on an ongoing basis. In order to accomplish these goals, the following are a few basic guidelines.

Basic Guidelines

- Eat breakfast every day, ideally shortly after waking up
- Eat a small meal every 2-3 hours
- Keep portion sizes small
- Have either fruit or vegetables at every meal
- Plan your meals every day

This is an example of an ideal meal plan:

Basic Mealtime Guideline		Ideal Meal
7:00 a.m.	Breakfast	Eggs, whole grain toast and an apple
9:30 a.m.	Mid-morning snack	30 cashews & pear
12:00 noon	Lunch	Salad with strips of chicken or turkey
3:00 p.m.	Mid-afternoon snack	20 almonds & orange
6:00 p.m.	Dinner	Baked salmon, broccoli, wild rice
8:30 p.m.	Evening snack	Large bowl of fresh strawberries

What is a portion?
The following is a general listing of serving sizes:
- 1 cup — cold cereal, veggies, berries
- ½ cup – legumes, beans, cooked grains, pasta, oatmeal
- yogurt – 6 ounces
- milk – 8 ounces
- eggs – 2
- lean protein – 4 ounces
- nuts – 20-30
- cheese – ¼ cup
- bread – 2 slices
- bagel – 1
- English muffin – 1
- Tortilla – 1
- Pita bread – 1
- Fruit – 1

Approved Foods
Most people come home and dive into whatever in the fridge is quickest and easiest to prepare. A good place to start is by stocking the kitchen with inherently healthy and easy-to-prepare foods. To help you prevent impulse buys, it is recommended that you shop on a full stomach and put together a complete grocery list before going to the store. To assist in developing your shopping list, the following is a

complete listing of approved foods, and suggestions for specific brands for the whole-grain products, because food companies can be pretty deceptive in their marketing efforts. Many so-called "whole grains" contain a lot of refined white flour, which sends insulin levels soaring.

You may notice that there are no approved beverages on this list; that is because there are none. If you only drink water, you can eliminate the 500 calories needed to create a deficit. According to the USDA, 10 to 14 percent of our daily calories come through beverages. Believe it or not, a large Starbucks Frappacino contains 670 calories. A 20-ounce bottle of soda or fruit juice contains 250 calories. Alcoholic drinks are even worse, because they lower testosterone levels. These drinks contain empty calories with no nutritional value. When you only drink water, you can consume more calories through food, avoid hunger pangs and give your body the nutrients it needs. If you want a daily caffeine boost, an occasional cup of green tea is fine because it is low in calories.

Another source of empty calories (and trans fat) is cooking oils and margarine. You should use olive oil or canola oil or coat pans with a non-stick spray or Benecol spread, which is plant based and has been found to inhibit cholesterol absorption. Benecol spread tastes good and can be used as a low-calorie butter substitute. Olive oil is the healthiest choice because it contains phytonutrients like polyphenols, which have been found to prevent both heart disease and cancer. Unfortunately, olive oil is not good for frying because it has a low smoke temperature. Canola oil has a neutral taste, heart-healthy monounsaturated fats and has a much higher smoke temperature.

Approved Foods

Low-fat Dairy Products	Select Fruits	Protein Containing Omega-3 Fatty Acids	Other Lean Proteins
Milk* Yogurt* Cottage cheese* String cheese* Mozzarella cheese* Swiss cheese* Ricotta cheese*	Apples Grapefruit Oranges Strawberries Blackberries Raspberries Blueberries Peaches Cranberries	Mackerel Tuna Herring Sardines Lake trout Salmon Halibut Sablefish Flax seeds Omega-3 fortified Eggs	Eggs Skinless chicken Fish All shellfish Turkey Whey powder Elk Deer Peanut butter* Ostrich Gator
Healthy High-Glycemic Carbs	Vegetables	Other Fruits	Other Protein Sources
Baked potatoes Bananas All types of melon Raisins Pineapple Mangos, grapes	All vegetables	All fruits	All nuts All beans All legumes
Whole Grains			
Breads Sara Lee Home-Style Wheat Milton's Healthy Whole Grain Thomas's New York Style Whole Wheat Bagels Wonder Stone Ground 100% Whole Wheat Matthews Whole Wheat English Muffins **Pasta** Hodgson Mill Whole Wheat Spaghetti De Cecco Whole Wheat Linguine Annie's Whole Wheat Shells and Cheddar Fantastic Whole Wheat Couscous **Oatmeal** Quaker Instant Oatmeal Quaker Quick Minute Oats		**Tortillas** Mission Low Carb tortillas Thomas' Sahara 100% Whole Wheat pita **Rice** Fantastic Brown Basmati Rice Uncle Ben's Instant Brown Rice Webman's Quick Cook Spanish Brown Rice Kraft Minute Instant Brown Rice **Cold Cereal** Post Raisin Bran Post Bran Flakes Kellogg's Shredded Wheat Wheat Chex Fiber One Wheaties Mother's Multi-Grain Cheerios Whole Foods Granola	
* In small portions and only products derived from free-range cattle.			

Cheat Days

"On the seventh day, thou shall cheat." So said Bill Phillips, a veritable god to more than two million individuals who have developed their best bodies using his system. Phillips advises all transformation aspirants to diet for six days and then cheat on the seventh, meaning that you can eat whatever you want, guilt-free. It does not mean that you can gorge yourself. Portion control and maintaining a calorie deficit are still overriding factors.

During the first four weeks of my first transformation program, I went off the deep end on my free day, eating lots of chips and cookies. The difference in how I felt the next day was pretty dramatic. I was sluggish and my muscles responded poorly during workouts. There is an old saying in the computer industry: "GIGO" Garbage In = Garbage Out. The human body works the exact same way. Once you have eaten clean for six days, then put garbage in on the seventh day, you can really see how important it is to maintain proper nutrition. Personally, I want my mind and body to perform at a peak level all the time, so I no longer ingest trans fat — ever. I still cheat on Sundays, usually with red meat or chocolate, but I try to keep the "cheating" in moderation. The virtues of taking a day off the diet are many, but you need to be smart about it. Do not waste your splurge on vanilla ice cream. On cheat days plan and prepare something special and really enjoy it.

Following is a full week of delicious meals you can make from the approved foods listing.

Top Six Breakfast Meals
1. Fresh trout and 2 eggs, 1 piece of whole grain toast, 1 tablespoon raspberry preserves, 1 glass of water.
2. Whole wheat toasted bagel with peanut butter and strawberry preserves, 1 glass of water.
3. Large bowl of oatmeal with blueberries, 1 cup of green tea.
4. Four egg whites scrambled, 1 piece of lean Canadian bacon, 1 piece of fruit, 1 cup of green tea.
5. Salmon omelet, 1 slice of whole-grain toast, 1 tablespoon of strawberry preserves, 1 glass of water.
6. Bowl of whole-grain cold cereal with milk, piece of select fruit.

Top Six Lunch Meals
1. Fresh romaine or spinach salad with a large variety of vegetables and lean meat — chicken, fish, shrimp or turkey. Avoid bacon bits, croutons, processed sliced meats, and all creamy mayonnaise-based dressings. Keep dressing on the side and dip fork into it prior to each bite. Some low-calorie dressings to consider include: Newman's Own Light Caesar Dressing, Hidden Valley Ranch Fat-Free, Emeril's Balsamic Vinaigrette.
2. Vegetable soup and a grilled chicken breast.
3. Tuna sandwich with tomatoes and cucumbers on whole wheat bread.
4. Chicken burrito with tomatoes, onions, olives, beans, peppers, mozzarella cheese in whole-wheat tortilla.
5. Baked turkey breast and Swiss cheese with favorite veggies in whole-wheat pita.
6. Salmon filet with three-bean salad.

Top Six Dinner Meals
1. Baked chicken breast, steamed spinach, baked sweet potato.
2. Broiled chicken with wild rice and Asian veggies — snow peas, water chestnuts.
3. Salmon filet, mixed veggies and brown rice.
4. Whole-wheat linguini with tomato sauce and shrimp with a salad on the side. Try the all-natural Lucini's pasta sauces.
5. Tuna noodle casserole with broccoli and mozzarella cheese.
6. Pizza — that's right, pizza is good for your diet if you follow this recipe: Get whole-wheat pizza dough from a health food store. Roll a thin crust onto a pizza pan; top with a cup of canned pizza sauce and a half-cup of low-fat mozzarella cheese. Load on the veggies: mushrooms, onions, peppers, zucchini, asparagus spears, whatever your favorites might be. You can also top with turkey pepperoni, which has the pepperoni taste you desire without artery-clogging fat. A 12" pan will make two ideal sized meals, so share with a friend.

Top Six Mid-Morning & Mid-Afternoon Snacks

1. An apple or banana with one large spoonful of peanut butter. Try Crazy Richard's Natural Chunky — roasted peanuts are the only ingredient.
2. A can of sardines or herring packed in water with one piece of select fruit.
3. Bran muffin and a glass of cold low-fat milk.
4. Join the "Breakfast Club" — have a bowl of whole-grain cereal using creamy vanilla soy protein instead of milk and top with blueberries.
5. An apple and 20 almonds.
6. Cantaloupe and yogurt — cut a cantaloupe in half, take out the seeds and pour in a 6-ounce serving of low-fat yogurt.

Top Six Soy Protein Shake Recipes

1. Strawberry-Banana Blast — 1 or 2 scoops strawberry soy protein, 1 cup fresh strawberries, 1 cup low-fat milk, 1 banana, 2 tbsps. flaxseed oil and ice blended.
2. Blueberry-Citrus Smoothie — 1 or 2 scoops vanilla soy protein, 1 cup fresh blueberries, 1 orange, 1 cup low-fat milk, 2 tbsps. flaxseed oil and ice blended.
3. Honey Dew Melon Smoothie — 1 or 2 scoops vanilla soy protein, 1 honeydew melon, 1 cup low-fat milk, 2 tbsps. of flaxseed oil and ice blended.
4. Chocolate-Peanut Butter Blast — 1 or 2 scoops chocolate soy protein, 1 heaping spoonful of peanut butter, 1 cup low fat milk, 2 tbsps. flaxseed oil and ice blended.
5. Blackberry-Oatmeal Blast — 1 or 2 scoops vanilla soy protein, 1 packet regular instant oatmeal, 1 cup fresh blackberries, 2 tbsps. flaxseed oil and ice blended.
6. The Classic — 1 or 2 scoops soy protein (any flavor), 1 cup cold low-fat milk in tumbler with sealable lid. Shake vigorously. Add 1 piece select fruit on the side. This is the easiest and most convenient recipe. I have a classic for my mid-morning and mid-afternoon snacks, only because I do not have access to berries or a blender.

8

THE POWER OF PURPOSE

In the Introduction I mentioned that during a Thanksgiving Day visit, my mother encouraged me to write a fitness book detailing the transformation program through which I had guided Charlie and Jim. That same day she also suggested I consider writing a book/program to help convicted felons end the repeat-offender cycle. I shared this thought with my roommate, Mike, who commented that he found it inspiring that, in spite of a life sentence, I was able to work toward achieving a goal and maintain a positive mental attitude almost every day. "If you could bottle that," he said, "you could help a lot of people in and out of prison." His words caused me to revisit the lessons I had learned from Viktor Frankl and Stephen Covey. Discovering purpose in life through serving others enabled me to defeat depression and turn my life around. The more I thought about it, the more I became motivated to share the things I had learned.

As a person who may never even get out of prison, the repeat-offender syndrome really bothers me. The institution where I am housed is a Reception Center (the first step for all convicted felons), so I see the same faces over and over again. I just could not comprehend how anybody who had been here once would jeopardize their freedom again by breaking the law. I interviewed these men, who were doing what I called "life on the installment plan," and it quickly became apparent that drug addiction was the big issue. By my estimation, 90 percent of repeat offenders and 75 percent of all men in prison committed drug-related crimes. If they were not selling or manufacturing drugs, they were either committing a crime to support their drug habit or were so high they did things they never would have done in a normal state of mind.

Dr. Chopra describes all addiction as a lack of exultation; meaning that something is missing from the person's life. From a mind-body medicine perspective the best way to treat any addiction is by helping addicts discover meaning in their lives, to replace the high of drugs with the exultation of purpose. As I considered this, I realized that the best way for me to help men end the repeat offender cycle was by helping them discover a meaningful career. I reasoned that if a man woke up every morning and said to himself, "I can't wait to get to work. I have the greatest job in the world," his life would be so filled with purpose that he wouldn't even consider using drugs or breaking the law.

I had experienced first-hand the power of meaning to transform a person's life. Frankl and Covey gave me the hope and expectation that my life still had value. The fact that I was incarcerated never really changed, but the meaning it held for me did. A new relationship with my adversity slowly developed and, in time, I discovered the most important work of my life. Now it was time for me to help others in the same way that my mentors had helped me.

I spent some time reviewing the lessons that inspired my own *purpose in life* transformation as well as a number of facts I had learned about behavioral medicine and personal coaching. In retrospect, I saw that the key to overcoming my suicidal depression was reconnecting with my passion for business. Developing Hooked On Health gave my life purpose. I also saw that the teachings of my health and fitness mentors had become ingrained in the form of a daily practice that enabled me to pursue that purpose every day, no matter how terrible the setback or what others felt about my chances of succeeding.

So I went to work on a second book/program called *Principles of Grace* that is designed to encourage readers to connect their deepest passion to a work they truly love and in so doing, discover a life that is meaningful and fulfilling. The book's message is succinctly described in the following passage from Dr. Wayne Dyer's inspirational bestseller *10 Secrets for Success & Inner Peace:*

> **The intuitive voice from within which says, "I love animals," or "I'm drawn to art," is there for a reason. Whatever it is that you love to do in life, I guarantee there is a way to make a living doing it while simultaneously serving others.**[1]

Shortly after starting to write *Principles of Grace,* my need to find a willing test subject became obvious. Insights gained from training Charlie and Jim were the very foundation of *Penitentiary Fitness*. It was my hope to find someone who would allow me to guide them through a purpose in life transformation. My months of searching were in vain.

Then one morning a young Hispanic gang member named Daniel Durland approached me while I was practicing yoga on the prison yard. He was curious about the ancient Hindu art, and I took the time to share my limited knowledge on the subject. As our conversation progressed, I mentioned my book about muscle development and fat loss. Daniel then told me about his own success with losing weight, stating that he went from 296 to 190 pounds in just five months. Curious, I pressed for details about his stunning transformation.

Here is what he told me: The first thing he did was trade all of his bread and butter for vegetables and his desserts (usually cake) for apples. Whenever he got hungry, he ate an apple. (Remember, apples are a select fruit that is 90 percent water and rich in the soluble fiber pectin, which makes you feel full longer.) He also traded in soft drinks for water. For exercise Daniel played handball (a high-intensity interval training sport) and did the exact same body-weight resistance training exercises that I do. He has a regular practice of writing down his workout plan and recording all results.

Daniel lost more than 100 pounds and confirmed practically everything I had written in the preceding chapters about diet and exercise. It was almost as if he had read my book; which was impossible because at this point it was neither finished, nor had I shown the early chapters to anyone. Equally as interesting is that earlier that same morning, I started writing a section titled "Expectations," in which I intended to give readers some idea of how long it would take them to achieve peak physical condition. Daniel's transformation was a perfect example, and he agreed to let me tell his story.

I decided to spend more time with Daniel. One afternoon while going for a walk I asked him where he learned so much about nutrition and exercise. He revealed that one of his previous cellmates named Bam Bam had taught him about weight loss. This was a surprising revelation because Bam Bam had gotten the information…from me! *Daniel had been doing my Hooked On Health program the whole time!* I immediately perceived that our chance encounter was a meaningful coincidence, or "synchronicity," a word created by pioneering psychoanalyst Carl Jung to describe when random events synchronize and fit together perfectly. In his book, *Synchronicity*, Jung describes the phenomenon:

> **Meaningful coincidences are thinkable as pure chance. But the more they multiply and the greater and more exact their correspondence is, the more their probability sinks and their unthinkability increases, until they can no longer be regarded as pure chance but, for lack of casual explanation, have to be thought of as *meaningful arrangements*.[2]**

Speaking on the same subject, Chopra proposes that coincidences (meaningful arrangements) are coded messages from God. In the audiotape series *The Spontaneous Fulfillment of Desire*, he states:

> **I do not believe in meaningless coincidence. I believe every coincidence is a message that requires our attention. By paying attention to life's coincidences you can learn to hear their message more clearly. And by understanding the forces that shape coincidence you can learn to influence those forces and create your own meaningful coincidences and take advantage of the opportunities they present.[3]**

Another highly respected health author, Dr. Bernie Siegal, writes, "Coincidence is God's way of remaining anonymous."[4] I have come to believe this is true. Early on in the development of Hooked On Health I learned to pay attention to synchronistic events and to discern their meaning. Invariably, these clues to the intention of the universe, to God's plan for my life, always led me in the right direction. Paying close attention to coincidences is one of the ways that human beings can tap into their own intuition.

Inspired by the synchronicity that Daniel had in fact been doing my Hooked On Health weight loss program all along, I decided to spend some time with him. I inquired about his criminal history. Sure enough, he was caught in the repeat-offender cycle, and drugs were a central issue. He has a history of using and selling illegal drugs. He was an ideal candidate for me to mentor and guide through my evolving *Principles of Grace* purpose in life program.

I told Daniel about Dr. Chopra's approach to drug addiction, and suggested that if he found a career where he was doing something that he loved every day, he could end the repeat-offender cycle. In time, he agreed to allow me to be his mentor. We discussed the things about which he was passionate, and the one subject that kept popping up was exercise. He loved to work out and also to motivate his "homeboys" to do so. Daniel was also intrigued by the science of muscle development and weight loss. Taken together, it was not too difficult to imagine Daniel being successful as a personal trainer and weight loss coach. He became enthusiastic about the idea.

With two years remaining on his sentence, Daniel enrolled in a mail-order personal fitness training course and prepared for his new career by guiding overweight inmates through the Hooked On Health program. He also developed a future vision of himself as the next Tai Bo, and made plans to create a *Penitentiary Fitness* exercise DVD based on workouts that convicts do during a lockdown.

As Daniel and I got to know one another, I learned that he had a tragic story of youth obesity. During the first five years of his life, Daniel's single mom struggled to make ends meet. Money was tight as she managed the difficult task of raising a toddler while working and attending school. They often were required to eat their meals at the local rescue mission. Eventually, they moved in with Daniel's grandmother, where Daniel had unlimited access to food for the first time in his young life. Daniel's grandmother stocked the cupboards with snacks and sweets, and after school he indulged in the foods that he never had access to before.

Daniel's mother completed her education and obtained a higher paying job. After many years of struggle, she was able to provide a better life for her son. The thing that young Daniel enjoyed the most was eating, and every day he begged his mother to take him to fast food restaurants. Like all mothers, she wanted to make her son happy, and their restaurant feasts became a time of joy. What Daniel's mother did not know, and what nutrition science is just beginning to teach us, is that fried foods and processed foods are addictive. They contain man-made chemicals that cause the body to release a neurotransmitter called "serotonin," which makes you feel really good. That's why junk foods are commonly referred to as "comfort foods" and the reason that people frequently reach for them when they are depressed or stressed out. The problem that arises with so-called comfort foods is as soon as the serotonin wears off, you get unnatural cravings for more comfort food. Despite the fact that you may not even need additional food, the mind sends out a hunger signal because it wants another "hit" of serotonin. Young Daniel became a serotonin food junkie. He was a victim of circumstance. After spending the first five years of his life on a sparse diet that was unsatisfying, he suddenly had access to foods that satisfied him in an important way. They made him feel good.

Daniel quickly became overweight, and by the time he entered middle school he was obese. There he encountered peer pressure for the first time in his life. He had difficulty making friends and felt like an outcast because of his weight. He was exposed to a number of humiliating social experiences. For example, his mother signed him up for a football league, hoping that the exercise would help him lose weight. At the weigh-in, he was told by the head coach that he was "too big to play with kids his own age." His experience at his first school dance was even worse. Daniel went shopping to buy the perfect outfit, got a haircut, and had high expectations, but none of the girls would dance with him. They called him fat and mocked him for even asking. A breaking point came after Daniel went with his mother to the state fair. The next day at school he was harassed by the other kids because he went with his mother and didn't have any friends.

Daniel began to get into fist fights with kids who made fun of him because of his weight, and started acting up in class. The school psychologist determined that he was antisocial and recommended that he be transferred to a school for kids with special needs called the "Individual Opportunities Program." Daniel wasn't antisocial. He was just a lonely kid who was desperate to fit in.

The Individual Opportunities Program was full of problem adolescents, and Daniel started hanging around with gang kids. In order to gain their acceptance, he began to use and sell drugs. Daniel quickly learned that when he had drugs, he attracted friends. People wanted to hang out with him, and he even started having girlfriends. Daniel soon made selling drugs a full-time career, which led to him committing other crimes, such as check fraud. Eventually, he was arrested and sent to prison. When Daniel was released, he returned to using and selling drugs. He was arrested again and again and again. For six years he repeated the cycle of committing crimes and going to prison. His life was an unmitigated disaster.

After learning about Daniel's tragic story of youth obesity, I became even more committed to helping him turn his life around. I tutored him on his personal fitness training course and continued to guide him through the *Principles of Grace* purpose in life program. Together we developed a step-by-step plan for his future and his new career as a weight loss transformation elicitor. I helped Daniel create an hour-long seminar called *The Amazing Weight Loss Formula*, which combined all of the most recent science on weight loss with his story of youth obesity. It was my great hope that he could earn a living and provide a much needed service to society by giving the seminar at high schools. Moreover, I hoped this noble mission would infuse his life with purpose and enable him to end his repeat-offender cycle.

Daniel practiced giving that seminar nearly every day for two years. He also completed his course to become a certified personal trainer. When his parole date arrived, Daniel seemed confident and poised to pursue his goals. Unfortunately, Daniel failed before he even got started. Shortly after his release on parole, Daniel was arrested for the fourth time in his life. At the age of only 27, he has returned to a life of incarceration.

I have related Daniel's story because it is informative on many levels. Daniel is a person who was obese his entire life. He thought that obesity was in his genes and that he would always be overweight. Yet, all he really needed was some advice about what foods to eat, what exercises to do, and to develop diligence about maintaining a negative energy balance. He went from 296 pounds to 190 pounds in just five months.

Daniel's experience with youth obesity is enlightening in that we can see just how destructive and addictive fast food and junk food really is. His story also reveals that junk food addiction and drug addiction are similar problems; both are frequently the result of depression. Overweight people who are depressed often turn to comfort foods because they turn on the neurochemicals that make them feel good, at least temporarily. Yet the quick fix never works. When the serotonin euphoria wears off, the junk food eater crashes and becomes even more depressed. It quickly becomes a vicious cycle in which out-of-balance brain chemicals cause intense junk food cravings and overeating, resulting in increased body fat. Fortunately, there is a solution: high-intensity exercise. Consider the following passage from Dr. Deepak Chopra's *Ageless Body — Timeless Mind:*

The brain mechanism that controls depression appears to lie within a class of neurochemicals called catecholamines. In depressed patients whose levels of catecholamines are abnormally low, healthy levels can be restored naturally through exercise.[4]

In a fascinating article titled "Running From Addiction" that appeared in *Maxim* magazine, writer Frank Owen describes how celebrities such as Robert Downey, Jr. and Owen Wilson overcame drug addiction by becoming workout junkies. He writes:

As researchers have come to learn, the drug high and the runner's high have a lot in common, namely brain chemicals, the mood-altering neurotransmitters that substances like cocaine, marijuana, and heroin mimic or activate.

Tests showed a dramatic increase in levels of endorphins in the blood of subjects who vigorously exercised... In addition to endorphins, researchers have identified other chemicals that are stimulated by intense exercise: dopamine, the substance that allows us to feel pleasure; serotonin, which acts as an antidepressant; and epinephrine, the body's natural amphetamine.[5]

Owen's article focused exclusively on the effectiveness of "the runner's high" to overcome drug abuse. Yet the therapeutic effect can be the same for depression and food addiction. If you replace the junk food with high-intensity exercise, the neurochemicals come into balance, and then depression and mood swings disappear. The result is vibrant physical and psychological health.

The other reason that I told Daniel's story is that I want people, especially parents, to become aware of the dire consequences of the scourge that is youth obesity. The Centers for Disease Control and Prevention estimate that one-third of American youths are overweight and 18 percent are obese. Overweight children are more likely to have behavioral and learning difficulties, and the low self-esteem likely to be formed during adolescence can last forever. Overweight kids suffer in many ways. They get teased and picked on by their peers. They spiral into depression, and then very bad things can happen to them. They could end up like Daniel — a bright, loving young boy who lashed out at his attackers and ended up in a school for troubled youths. Such schools are a breeding ground for future criminals and led Daniel to a life of crime. For other obese kids it can be even worse. They often turn to drugs to ease their psychological pain, and some even attempt suicide.

In the process of helping Daniel develop *The Amazing Weight Loss Formula* seminar, I became attached to the mission of helping prevent youth obesity. Following his bitter failure, I decided to continue pursuing that mission by transforming the seminar into *The Amazing Weight Loss Formula* audio book, and making it available from my website, JBarrettHawkins.com as a free download. The audio book contains everything that I have learned about losing weight, along with Daniel's story of youth obesity. I have also instituted a program that allows people to tell everyone on their buddy list about the free audio book by e-mailing online postcards. I want to encourage readers of this book to visit the website and download this free audio book as a means of reinforcing everything you have learned from *Penitentiary Fitness,* and also to use of e-postcard system to tell your friends about the program.

Daniel's failure also exposed the shortcomings of the *Principles of Grace* purpose in life program I was developing. Nothing motivates me more than failure. I dedicated myself to reading every book I could get my hands on concerning purpose in life and achieving one's ambitions. I read books written by personal coaches, executive coaches, spiritual masters, modern mystics, peak performance experts, and success strategists. With each book I took copious notes, distilling all of the best ideas, insights, advice, and success secrets into a program of my own. The result is *Principles of Grace,* a book loaded with wisdom, that will help people transform their dreams into reality. Many of the book's techniques can be applied to the pursuit of one's health and fitness goals. Therefore, this chapter concludes with suggestions for staying inspired and motivated.

FIVE TIPS FOR ONGOING INSPIRATION AND MOTIVATION

#1   Connect With Your Power of Purpose — Spend some time alone to contemplate why you want to get into shape. Maybe you want to be more attractive, improve your health, or have more energy to achieve your goals in life. Getting in touch with why you want to get into better shape is the most important step in any weight loss or fitness program. This is your power of purpose. Once you develop the ability to tap into that power on an ongoing basis, you can accomplish feats that you never dreamed possible.

#2   Set Audacious Long-term Goals & Achievable Short-term Objectives — If you knew beyond a shadow of a doubt that you could not fail in the pursuit of your health and fitness goals, what would you want to accomplish? Lose 100 pounds? Reverse your diabetes? Or perhaps develop a physique like a fitness model? The philosopher Goethe said: "Boldness has genius, power, and magic in it." And so it does. Aspire to your highest potential. Then identify the steps you will be required to take to get there and make a list of short-term objectives. If your audacious goal is to lose 100 pounds, list your daily objectives: 1) eliminate man-made junk foods, 2) eat five or six small meals, 3) walk 10,000 steps, 4) one hour of high-intensity exercise, and 5) get a good night's sleep. Set short-term goals such as losing a *minimum* of five pounds every month.

#3   Reaffirm Your Purpose & Goals With An Action Statement — Get a handful of 3" x 5" index cards. On each of them write 1) the reason why you want to get into top shape, 2) your audacious goal, and 3) a specific deadline for accomplishing your objective. Then make multiple copies of your action statement and place it everywhere: your nightstand, refrigerator, bathroom mirror, computer, car dashboard, wallet or purse. Connect with the statement first thing in the morning, prior to bedtime, and throughout the day. Don't just read your action statement; truly connect with your mission by visualizing the desired results and by expressing the powerful emotions of achieving your goal. In time, your action statement will become a belief statement. Once you believe that you can accomplish your goal, and are willing to take the necessary actions on a daily basis, then you will surely achieve your desired outcome.

#4   Develop A Strong Support Team — No matter what your goals in life are, you will always get there faster with the help of people who care about your success. With a fitness or weight loss objective, you'll want to enlist the help of a workout partner, an accountability partner, and the people you live with. A workout partner will ensure that you don't miss any workouts and will push you to train at higher levels of intensity. Daily contact via phone calls, e-mails, and text messaging with an accountability partner will help both of you stay focused on your goals. Finally, the people who you live with must maintain the same healthy diet as you, and agree to never bring processed junk food into your home.

#5   <u>Commit To Ongoing Personal Development</u> — Subscribe to health and fitness magazines such as *Muscular Development, Men's Fitness, Muscle Media, Flex, Prevention, Muscle & Fitness, Shape, Men's Health,* or *Maximum Fitness,* which are full of motivating articles. Read at least one health, fitness, or weight loss book every month. Listen daily to inspirational audio programs by experts such as Anthony Robbins, Jack Canfield, Wayne Dyer, Stephen Covey, or Denis Waitley, among others. Visit my website, JBarrettHawkins.com and download *The Amazing Weight Loss Formula* audio book free of charge. Make a commitment to listen to it once a week for motivation and to reinforce the action plan you will be employing to fulfill your aspirations.

WORKOUT PLANS

The *Hooked On Health* training system consists of six separate phases, each of which is a distinctly different workout. Which phases you use, as well as how many weeks you use them, will be predicated on your current level of fitness and your overall objective. A woman who is 100 pounds overweight and a professional male bodybuilder who is seeking new growth can both benefit; however, the workout plan must be tailored to their specific needs. Following is an outline of each phase and a variety of workout plans based on various individual objectives.

Phase 1 consists of a 20-minute total body resistance training workout that will be performed on Monday, Wednesday and Friday and one hour of high-intensity interval training sports activities on Saturday and Sunday.

Phase 2 consists of two separate 45-minute "Walk in Nature" resistance training workouts: one for upper body, one for lower body, that will be alternated on Monday, Wednesday and Friday, and one hour of high-intensity interval training sports activities on Saturday and Sunday.

Phase 3 consists of two 45-minute "Peak Performance" resistance training workouts: one for upper body, one for lower body that will be alternated on Monday, Wednesday and Friday, and a workout that combines sprinting (the absolute best high-intensity interval training exercise) with yoga stretching on Tuesday, Thursday and Saturday.

Phase 4 consists of two 45-minute "Peak Performance" resistance training workouts: Push — for chest, shoulders, triceps; and Pull — for back and biceps, to be alternated on Monday, Wednesday and Friday. Two "combo" workouts that incorporate sprinting with resistance training of one body part: legs with sprinting or abs with sprinting to be alternated on Tuesday, Thursday and Saturday. *Phases 5 and 6* are based on advanced double-session training methods. Phase 5, the bulking phase, is strictly for men who want to develop enormous muscles. Phase 6, the cutting phase, requires two short but intense workouts: a 30-minute resistance training session in the morning and a 20-minute session of guerrilla cardio in the evening. Phase 6 is a training split of four days on and one day off. Extra diet recommendations are offered to burn the last of your body fat.

	Week	Exercise Plan
Workout Plan A is for male or female who wants to lose body fat and develop a sleek, muscular physique, but has a hectic schedule and limited time to work out during the week.	1	Phase 1 Beginner
	2	Phase 1 Beginner
	3	Phase 1 Beginner
	4	Phase 1 Beginner
	5	Phase 1 Intermediate
	6	Phase 1 Intermediate
	7	Phase 1 Intermediate
	8	Phase 1 Intermediate
	9	Phase 1 Advanced
	10	Phase 1 Advanced
	11	Phase 1 Advanced
	12	Phase 1 Advanced
	Week	Exercise Plan
Workout Plan B is for male or female who is moderately (up to 30 pounds) overweight and out of shape and who wants to develop a sleek, muscular physique, or a person not necessarily overweight but has not been exercising and would like to achieve peak physical condition.	1	Phase 1
	2	Phase 1
	3	Phase 2
	4	Phase 2
	5	Phase 3
	6	Phase 3
	7	Phase 4
	8	Phase 4
	9	Phase 4
	10	Phase 4
	11	Phase 6
	12	Phase 6

	Week	Exercise Plan
Workout Plan C is for a male or female who is overweight (over 30 pounds) and who wants to lose weight and have a sleek, muscular physique. Individuals who are extremely overweight may require four additional weeks of training to achieve their goals.	1	Phase 2
	2	Phase 2
	3	Phase 2
	4	Phase 2
	5	Phase 3
	6	Phase 3
	7	Phase 3
	8	Phase 3
	9	Phase 4
	10	Phase 4
	11	Phase 4
	12	Phase 4
	13	Phase 6
	14	Phase 6
	15	Phase 4
	16	Phase 4

	Week	Exercise Plan
Workout Plan D is for male bodybuilders who have lifted weights for a minimum of three months consecutively and who are looking for new ways to stimulate massive growth.	1	Phase 4
	2	Phase 4
	3	Phase 4
	4	Phase 4
	5	Phase 5
	6	Phase 5
	7	Phase 5
	8	Phase 5
	9	Phase 6
	10	Phase 6
	11	Phase 6
	12	Phase 6

WARMING UP AND COOLING DOWN

Before performing any of the workouts outlined in upcoming chapters, you must spend between 5 and 10 minutes warming up your body. The purpose of the warm-up is to prepare your heart, your muscles and joints for intense training. The objective is to slowly elevate your heart rate and stimulate blood flow, which in turn increases muscle temperature and lubricates the joints. A proper warm-up routine consists of five minutes of low-intensity aerobic activity (jogging, skipping rope, jumping jacks), followed by gentle stretching that targets the muscles you will be working, and finally two light sets if you are doing resistance training. Muscles, tendons and ligaments all become much more pliable and responsive when warm. If you skip the warm-up, you run the risk of injury to muscles, joints and even the heart. I've actually read accounts of individuals having heart attacks because they put too much strain on the heart before it was ready.

High-intensity resistance training places incredible demands on the mind as well as the body. For optimal results, it is important to warm up your brain. Preparing your central nervous system for activity is just as important as preparing your muscles. One way to do this brain warming is by cultivating a positive mental attitude while warming up your body. If you dread the workouts going in, you will not get the results you desire. Negative attitudes lead to negative behavior. Instead of thinking about how hard the workouts are, spend time concentrating on the results for which you will be striving. You can also focus on the body parts you will be training as well as specific goals for each workout.

A pre-workout routine can also help eliminate outside distractions. Whatever is going on in your life, either positive or negative, needs to be left behind when you get ready to exercise.[1] That's the only way you can achieve optimal results. My training sessions are a most important part of my life. It's the one time in my day I can escape and relieve the stress that comes with living in a cage.

I use visualization and positive self-talk during my aerobic warm-up to create mind-body harmony and harness my intensity. I visualize myself doing a particular exercise with explosive force, feeling the motion of the muscle and experiencing the burn of a maximum intensity set. Visualization excites the same neurological pathways as actual performance and awakens cellular intelligence.[2] At the same time, you can empower yourself with positive affirmations such as, "Today's going to be my best workout ever," or "I feel like I can conquer the world." Believe it or not, these techniques can really psych you up and empower you to exercise harder, all of which lead to better results.

Cooling Down
Like warming up before a workout, cooling down afterwards is important. When you do a resistance-training workout, your muscles become engorged with blood; this is good because "the pump" is associated with muscle growth, but it can also be dangerous, because when you stop working out the blood pools in your muscles, meaning there is less blood and oxygen returning to your heart. To eliminate the possibility of a post-workout heart attack, you need to get circulating some of the oxygen that is in the blood that has pooled in the muscle. A brisk five-minute walk or some light aerobics will get the job done, but I prefer doing yoga.

Yoga stretching after a resistance-training workout enhances muscle recovery, reduces soreness and maximizes flexibility. Yoga can also shut down cortisol and enhance weight loss. A study published in *Alternative Therapies* found that individuals' cortisol levels dropped following a yoga session. The researchers also concluded that those who practiced yoga regularly lost more weight than those who did not.[3] From a muscle development perspective this result is significant, because high-intensity resistance training is a stress that causes the body to release cortisol, and cortisol causes the breakdown of muscles and inhibits their uptake of nutrients. Cortisol has also been found to blunt testosterone's muscle-building actions. Since resistance training causes testosterone levels to rise, a post-workout, cortisol-killing yoga session can be viewed as a testosterone booster.

After a resistance-training workout, I recommend going through the Sun Salutation a minimum of four times. Then, stretch the body part you trained twice, holding the posture for four deep breaths on the first stretch and eight deep breaths on the second; four deep breaths take about 30 seconds and eight take around 60 seconds. After aerobic exercise I recommend that you do a full 20-minute routine of fixed postures. After a cardio workout — particularly those you will find in Chapters 11 to 13 — the entire body is warm and receptive to being stretched. I usually do a 20-minute routine of fixed postures consisting of every stretch found in the yoga series.

Yoga Stretching

A regular yoga practice can deliver a remarkable range of health benefits. Perhaps the most important benefit of yoga is transmitting oxygen into every cell of your body. In fact, if cells do not get enough oxygen, they die.

Dr. Otto Warburg, Nobel Prize winner and director of the Max Planck Institute of Cell Physiology, studied the effects of oxygen on cells. He was able to turn normal, healthy cells into malignant cells simply by lowering the amount of oxygen available to them. Thus, the quality of your health is directly related to the quality of the life of your cells.[4] Fully oxygenating your system also increases circulation, which bathes muscles, joints, connective tissue and internal organs in fresh blood; this in turn has a cosmetic effect as skin becomes softer, shinier and smoother (fewer wrinkles).[5]

According to Godfrey Devereau, author of the insightful book *Dynamic Yoga,* "The ancient yogis began their practice with the Sun Salutation, a flowing sequence of poses designed to warm up their body and awaken the latent power and intelligence of every muscle cell. Each of the poses challenges a different network of cells in the tendons, ligaments, muscles and even the internal organs."[6] These poses create an environment for optimal blood flow, supplying the cells with oxygen, glucose, minerals and energy. As the cells become activated, the nerve impulses flow more freely and the mind-body connection realizes its full potential. Devereau instructs:

> **The body must be awakened slowly. The systematic posture sequencing of the Sun Salutation is based on the natural laws of physical movement, enabling you to gradually stretch the**

muscles and joints, while at the same time awakening their somatic intelligence. For those just beginning a yoga practice, you should progress slowly. If you push or pull yourself into painful positions before your body is ready, you will probably cause injury. New neural pathways must be established between the spine and muscle cells, and this takes time. Be patient. Eventually, through the repetition of daily practice, you will find yourself performing the poses effortlessly.[7]

Another fantastic yoga resource is Gary Kraftsow's *Yoga for Wellness.* Kraftsow's book describes *viniyoga,* which delivers a remarkable range of health benefits. He writes:

Viniyoga is a practice that includes both repetitive movements of the body into and out of postures and the holding of particular postures for extended periods of time. Through alternate stretching and contracting, repetition increases circulation to the larger superficial skeletal muscles, making them stronger and more flexible. Thus, repetition prepares us for holding postures for extended periods of time with minimal resistance.[8]

When you hold a posture, tension on the muscles increases. At first, this holding causes the spinal cord to instruct the muscles to shorten as a protective mechanism to prevent them from being overstretched. It takes about 10 seconds for the brain and spinal cord to realize that the stretch is safe. At this point, the tightness you feel of the muscle shortening will disappear and the muscle will stretch more easily. It is during the next 20 to 40 seconds that the stretch releases tension from the body and delivers its other health benefits. With the holding postures it is essential not to bounce while stretching. Bouncing causes a reflex contraction that can lead to injury.

The most significant benefits of yoga (as opposed to stretching) lie in our ability to link the conscious mind to the unconscious rhythms of the body. We accomplished this through breathing. In the moving Sun Salutation postures, the breath leads the body and synchronizes the movement — we inhale when the front of the body opens and exhale when it closes. Yoga becomes a form of meditation when you stop thinking and focus all of your mental attention on the sensations in your body during inhalation and exhalation. At first you will feel the air moving in and out of your lungs, but as you connect your mind to the stretch and follow the breath you can feel the freshly oxygenated blood pulsating through your muscles.

Personally, I start each day with a short Morning Practice yoga routine that takes about 10 minutes. I begin by reading my own mission statement and thinking deeply about the goals I aspire to achieve. In the Eastern yogic tradition, this is known as a "sutra," a seed in consciousness that will expand my awareness throughout the day, enabling me to zero in on my objectives.[*] Next, I do the Sun Salutation a minimum of four times, clearing my mind of all thought and focusing my mental attention solely on the breath. Then I do a series of fixed postures, holding each pose from the Sun Salutation for four deep breaths. A Morning Practice is a great way to awaken the body and sharpen the mind before beginning your day.

Morning Practice

Sun Salutation x 4   Yoga Series 601-611, 4 deep breaths per posture   (see page 158)

20-Minute Yoga Routine

Yoga Series 601-623, 4 deep breaths per posture   Yoga Series 601-623, 8 deep breaths per posture   (see page 158-161)

---

[*] If you would like to learn more about expanding your consciousness and achieving your goals in life, visit the author's website, www.JBarrettHawkins.com, and read a sample chapter from his next book, *Principles of Grace: The Teachings of the Medicine Man.*

11

LOCKDOWN: THE 20-MINUTE TOTAL BODY WORKOUT

The most common excuse people give for not exercising is that they simply do not have the time. In response to this dilemma, I have designed a 20-minute total body workout that (a) revs up your metabolism by building muscle mass; (b) improves cardiovascular fitness and strengthens the heart, and (c) incorporates core body stretching to increase flexibility. So shelve that excuse, because you can get all of the necessary health benefits in one intense fat-burning routine.

As we learned earlier, high-intensity interval training is the best type of aerobic exercise for shedding fat. The 20-Minute Total Body Workout uses an interval-training concept known as circuit training to develop cardiovascular fitness and build muscle. You will perform a series of body-weight resistance training exercises — one pull exercise for back and biceps; one core training series to work your abs and lower back; one push exercise to hit the chest, shoulders and triceps; one leg exercise and one set of cardio push-ups to target your cardiovascular system. These five exercises are performed back to back with no rest between sets; that is one circuit. You will be doing four consecutive circuits with no rest, for a grand total of 20 sets. The exercise series is quick, efficient and intense.

Full-body circuit training is particularly effective for strengthening the cardiovascular system. Most heart attacks are caused by plaque blockages that develop in blood vessels. With this regimen, the training includes the back first, then the mid-section, followed by the chest and shoulders, then the legs and finishes up with an exercise that works every muscle in the body. When you exercise a particular muscle, it becomes engorged with blood. Then, when you switch to another muscle, the blood rushes in that direction. This type of training "exercises" your capillaries, the small blood vessels that deliver oxygen, amino acids and hormones to your muscles. The workout clears the pipes, so to speak, decreasing plaque buildup and the potential for blockages, and will also increase the number of working capillaries, allowing better nutrient transfer.

To add flexibility benefits and strengthen your core muscles — the abs and lower back — a notoriously effective Pilates routine called the Series of Fives is incorporated. Joseph H. Pilates was one of the early pioneers of mind-body medicine. During the 1920's he developed a fitness program that combined mind, body and spirit. The Pilates method is used by numerous professional sports teams. The Pilates exercises develop what has become known as the body's core — the entire mid-section of the body. When this core group of muscles is properly trained, not only will it help you create a great physique, it will also prevent lower back injuries.

The 20-Minute Total Body Workout will enable you to achieve a high level of fitness because it is designed to tax both your aerobic and your anaerobic systems. The key to the routine's success is the fifth exercise in the circuit — the cardio push-up. In addition to working every muscle in the body, this indigenous prison exercise will put great demands on your cardiovascular system.

After completing a set of cardio push-ups, you immediately return to the first four exercises, which are far less demanding aerobically; this is called an active recovery phase, in which your cardio system is forced to recover while still under stress. The fourth and final time through the circuit you add what Bill Phillips calls a "high point" — in this case an extra minute of cardio push-ups. The intensity and lactic acid burn is off the charts, but when you push through the pain, you will experience a tremendous spike in your metabolism.

According to John P. Hussman, author of the extraordinary thesis, *Why the Body-for-Life Program Works*:

> **This kind of interval training contributes greatly to your aerobic performance, and has been found to improve the neurological pathways your body uses for recruiting muscle fibers. There is a whole list of metabolic benefits that comes from this approach, including higher lactate tolerance, greater capillary density, increased fat-burning enzymes and transfer agents, expansion of muscle glycogen stores, and increase in mitochondria (the parts of the cell that produce energy).[1]**

The 20-Minute Total Body Workout was inspired by Phillips' 20-Minute Aerobic Solution. During times when the prison was "locked down" (I was confined to an 8' by 10' cell), I had to find a way to deal with the stress. Imagine waking up to the sound of rap music blaring, people yelling and screaming like lunatics and a cellmate defecating only a few feet away. It almost drove me insane. Bill's Solution became my saving grace. I rolled out of my bunk, drank a glass of water and then got right to it. I tortured my body for 20 minutes and the environmentally induced stress magically disappeared. The ensuing endorphin rush lifted my spirits and I spent the rest of the day working on Hooked On Health or my various writing projects. Bill's Solution focuses exclusively on cardio. This workout is different because it also emphasizes muscle development.

For individuals who choose to do this routine, it is recommended that you perform it first thing in the morning before breakfast. Start your day with a personal victory over self and you will develop a mindset that will lead to more victories throughout the day.[2] Your energy level will be much higher and you will feel good about yourself, because you have taken care of the one important thing you never have time for — your health. You will also burn more fat. Research shows that exercising first thing in the morning in a fasted state forces the body to tap into fat stores to fuel the workout.

I was able to do the 20-Minute Total Body Workout every day as aerobic training because my body had already adapted to the exercises. For those of you just starting out, you will get an aerobic workout and a muscle-building workout. Provided are three different exercise plans — beginner, intermediate and advanced. Time-starved individuals can complete a 12-week transformation program by spending four weeks at each level, enabling the development of a high level of fitness; however, it is not enough to develop your best physique. The human body is incredibly adaptive and at some point (different for everyone) this will also become just an aerobic exercise for you. At that juncture you will move on to the workouts outlined in the following chapters if you want to continue developing your physique.

The Morning Practice is an ideal warm-up for this routine, but if really pressed for time you can skip it because during the first circuit you will only be doing 50 percent of your maximum capacity, and that will suffice for a warm-up. On the second circuit you will raise the level of intensity to 75 percent of maximum capacity. On the third and fourth circuits you need to push the intensity envelope, doing as many repetitions of each exercise as you can handle. These exercises will be challenging your muscles in ways they have never before been challenged. Take it easy with the first two circuits. If your muscles are not warm enough, you can quite easily injure yourself.

You should begin to sweat after the second circuit and be breathing really hard after the third. The fourth circuit is the most important and most difficult. For optimal results, you need to bring maximum effort, maximum intensity, to each of the last two circuits. When you hit your high point — your second set of cardio push-ups — your muscles and lungs should be searing from pain. That's the lactic acid buildup. If you can gut it out for a full two minutes, you will be rewarded with a wonderful endorphin high that will leave you feeling fantastic.

Since there are three different levels of intensity (beginner, intermediate and advanced) and four circuits in each that also need varying levels of cardiovascular intensity, I had to tailor the cardio push-up accordingly. Hence, there are five different levels of cardio push-ups.

Cardio push-up I combines a toe touch, knee raise, squat thrust and push-up.
Cardio push-up II combines a knee raise, squat thrust and push-up.
Cardio push-up III combines a squat thrust, push-up and jump squat.
Cardio push-up IV combines a squat thrust, two push-ups and a jump squat.
Cardio push-up V combines a squat thrust, three push-ups and a jump squat.

Number III is the basic cardio push-up. When you eliminate the jump squat and add a knee raise, the level of intensity decreases, and when you add both a toe touch and a knee raise, it becomes even easier. The intensity level increases when you add a second or third push-up to each repetition. (See Chapter 16 for precise instructions.)

Your current level of fitness and muscle soreness will determine the number of weeks that you stay in each level (beginner, intermediate or advanced). When your muscles stop getting sore, it is time to move up. Also, it is best to not spend any more than four weeks at any one level, because your muscles will adapt quickly and require new stimulus to continue growing. Ideally, you should do the 20-Minute Total Body Workout every Monday, Wednesday and Friday; however, if you have not been exercising at all, your muscles may not recover fast enough during the first two weeks. If you are sore when you wake up Wednesday morning, do not do the routine. Your muscles should fully recover before you blast them again. Thus, you may have to do only two sessions (Monday and Friday) the first couple of weeks. Even if you are extremely out of shape, your muscles will adapt quickly, and by week three you should be recovering in less than 48 hours. For consistency and to reduce soreness, it is recommended that you do the morning practice stretching routine at the same time on Tuesday and Thursday.

To round out this workout plan, you should spend a full hour both Saturday and Sunday training your cardio system by playing sports or engaging in an activity that you truly enjoy (See page 31 for a list of activities that employ the high-intensity training principles.) If you have a busy, hectic life, these may very well be the two most important hours of your week. The time you spend in play will enhance your overall sense of well-being and recharge your energy system, thus making you more effective in all phases of your life.

Phase 1: Training Split

Day	Workout	Body Parts Trained
Monday	Resistance	Total Body
Tuesday	Off	
Wednesday	Resistance	Total Body
Thursday	Off	
Friday	Resistance	Total Body
Saturday	Aerobic	Cardio System
Sunday	Aerobic	Cardio System

The 20-Minute Total Body Workout

	Beginner	Intermediate	Advanced
Cycle #1			
1	Low-intensity Pull-ups	Low-intensity Pull-ups	Curl Pull-ups
2	Pilates (3)	Pilates (5)	Pilates (7-10)
3	Low-intensity Push-ups	Classic Push-ups	Dips
4	Jumping Jacks	Squats	Squats
Cycle #2			
1	Low-intensity Pull-ups	Static Hang	Curl Pull-ups
2	Pilates (3)	Pilates (5)	Pilates (7-10)
3	Low-intensity Push-ups	Classic Push-ups	Dips
4	Jumping Jacks	Alternating Lunges	Mountain Climbers
5		Cardio Push-up I	Cardio Push-up III
Cycle #3			
1	Low-intensity Pull-ups	Static Hang	Curl Pull-ups
2	Pilates (3)	Pilates (5)	Pilates (7-10)
3	Low-intensity Push-ups	Classic Push-ups	Deep Stretch Push-ups
4	Squats	Mountain Climbers	Jump Squats
5	Cardio Push-up I	Cardio Push-up II	Cardio Push-up IV
Cycle #4			
1	Low-intensity Pull-ups	Static Hang	Curl Pull-ups
2	Pilates (3)	Pilates (5)	Pilates (7-10)
3	Low-intensity Push-ups	Classic Push-ups	Deep Stretch Push-up
4	Squats	Mountain Climbers	One legged Squats
5	Cardio Push-up II	Cardio Push-up III	Cardio Push-up V
6		Cardio Push-up III	Cardio Push-up V

Training Tips and Insights:

- The Cardio push-ups are performed for one minute or until failure, whichever comes first.
- The exercises flow from one exercise to the next without any rest in between.
- The numbers in parenthesis represent the number of repetitions for each of the five Pilates exercises.

The only piece of equipment you may need to purchase for this workout is a pull-up bar. One of the sturdiest bars is the Door Gym, which fits in any doorway and requires no mounting hardware.

12

WALK IN NATURE WORKOUTS

When playing football in high school our coach made us "hit the lines" as a form of punishment whenever a player made a mental error in practice. This order meant that we had to jog the length of the field and back while dropping to the ground to do five push-ups at every white line. Since there is a line every five yards, we did 40 sets of five push-ups in a short period of time; it was indeed punishing. I flashed back to this one day as I watched a couple of convicts doing sets of push-ups while walking the track, and it occurred to me to develop a series of workouts that could be done while going for a walk.

According to Deepak Chopra, an early-morning walk in the sunshine and fresh air is one of the best things that we can do to promote health. The sights, sounds, tastes, smells and even touch of nature are healing; they nourish the body, mind and soul. In fact, everything in the environment that we place our attention on is *metabolized* into a new form of who we are. We literally *digest* the universe through our sensory organs.[1] Prior to outlining the Walk in Nature Workouts, a brief look at what modern science has to say about this phenomenon seems in order. This look, which was adapted from Dr. Deepak Chopra and Dr. David Simon's audio series *Training the Mind — Healing the Body,* will help us gain a basic understanding of how we can improve our physiology through forming a connection with nature.

Taste is the easiest to understand. When we eat a steak, for example, the body breaks it down into amino acids, glucose, fats, minerals, etc., then rebuilds these elements into your heart, lungs, muscles, bones, etc. and eliminates what it does not need. The human body is constantly renewing itself. In the course of a year, 98 percent of the atoms in your body will be *exchanged* with the environment.[2] This is why it is wise to rely on nature for your carbohydrates and why foods containing trans fat are so harmful. Since trans fat is a man-made substance not found in nature, our system does not recognize or digest it well and so stores it as fat.

Sound is another one to which it is fairly easy to relate. If you have a favorite type of music, just hearing it can lift your spirits. When you *ingest* the music you enjoy, the body *metabolizes* the sound and produces endorphins — the feel-good hormones. Research shows that music influences a number of physiological functions including blood pressure, heart rate and brain waves, to name a few. Music therapy is commonly used in clinics to treat a variety of medical conditions.[3]

Sight also has a profound influence on physiological processes. Research indicates that brain wave patterns, blood pressure and heart rate are different when a person takes in the beauty of nature — a rainbow, a waterfall or ocean waves crashing ashore — versus an urban scene — traffic jams, parking lots, brick buildings.[4] If you see a homeless person in the street, the emotions you experience and the chemical changes in your body will be different than if you are watching children play in the park.

Smell is perhaps the most fascinating of our sensory organs, because certain odors can cause changes in our bodies even below the level of our conscious awareness. One poignant example is when you encounter a dead animal or someone else's vomit. The smell immediately sets off physiological responses such as nausea. Contrast this reaction with the scent of pine trees or flowers, and you can easily see the positive effects of being in nature.

Touch is best illustrated through the amazing physiological changes that occur as the result of massage. Dr. Tiffany Fields of the Touch Research Institute at the University of Miami Medical School has demonstrated that massage stimulates the vagus nerve, which causes the body to release the mood-elevating neuro-transmitter serotonin. An example of changes that occur when touching nature can be illustrated through a study that found walking barefooted in grass calms anxious children.[5] You can also relate to swimming in the ocean or the cooling sensation of a breeze on a hot summer's day.

The tastes, sounds, sights, smells and touches of nature create positive physiological changes in human biochemistry. Thus, it stands to reason that our exercise sessions will be more effective if done at the beach, in the mountains, or simply while taking a walk in the park. There is nothing that I love more than to watch the early-morning sunshine stream through the misty dew and cast shadows over the mountains near where I work out. One of the best things about body-weight resistance training is that you do not have to pay to go to a gym. The training is an opportunity to commune with nature — to bring the fruits of the universe into your body. While this experience may not necessarily lead to less fat or bigger muscles, science has repeatedly demonstrated that it leads to better overall health.

The basic concept of these routines is that you will go for a walk in a setting that you like and stop occasionally to do a body-weight resistance training exercise. During the rest intervals you will continue walking while placing your mental attention and your senses on the beauty of nature. Try to really experience the environment: notice the shapes of the trees, the touch of the earth, the freshness in the air or the vibrant colors of a flower. If you are doing these routines with a partner, the rest intervals are a great time to discuss your training goals and reinforce the action plan you will be employing to reach your objectives. Most parks have some type of pull-up bar, which will be needed for the upper body workouts. With these exercises it is also wise to walk, say, 30 yards and back, between sets. This brisk walking between exercises constitutes an "active recovery" phase that enables you to burn more fat.

Your current level of fitness will determine the rep count and the exercise tempo. Ideally, you should do between 6 to 12 repetitions on the upper body exercises and 12 to 25 repetitions on the leg exercises. Legs respond much better to higher reps. It is important to hit the muscles from multiple angles, and for this reason we perform a number of different exercises. Begin with a tempo of three seconds down (negative) and one second up (positive). Slow down the negative portion on all exercises and focus your mind on the muscle fibers, then explode up on the positive and flex the muscle hard at the top. You want to be near failure on the final repetition of each set. If an exercise is too easy, you can increase the intensity by slowing down the tempo. Research from numerous studies indicates that super-slow repetition training increases muscular tension and produces greater gains in strength. A patient tempo, with the negative portion taking eight seconds to perform, is a great way to increase the intensity of a resistance training exercise. To be radical you can stop for a couple of seconds at mid-repetition a few times, descending in staggered fashion. When you use super-slow repetition training it is important to breathe normally throughout the movement. As you become more comfortable with these exercises, you will get a "feel" for the tempo needed to approach failure on your final rep.

The Walk in Nature Workouts are longer than those described in Chapter 11 (40 minutes as opposed to 20 minutes) and the resistance training is more intense. However, these workouts do not tax the cardio system. This training split alternates upper-body and lower-body resistance workouts on Monday, Wednesday and Friday. Your days off will be Tuesday and Thursday, and you will get aerobics on the weekend by playing sports or engaging in other high-intensity interval training activities that you enjoy. With this workout plan you will do six upper body and six lower body resistance-training sessions over a four-week period. In each session you will be doing five different exercises. The number of sets and the amount of rest between sets are the variables that can be used to slightly raise the intensity level with each workout.

Phase 2 : Training Split

	Week 1	Week 2	Week 3	Week 4
Monday	Upper body (1)	Lower Body (2)	Upper Body (4)	Lower Body (5)
Tuesday	Off	Off	Off	Off
Wednesday	Lower Body (1)	Upper Body (3)	Lower Body (4)	Upper Body (6)
Thursday	Off	Off	Off	Off
Friday	Upper Body (2)	Lower Body (3)	Upper Body (5)	Lower Body (6)
Saturday	Cardio	Cardio	Cardio	Cardio
Sunday	Cardio	Cardio	Cardio	Cardio

Training Tips and Insights:

- *Focus on Form*: In the beginning, do not be too concerned with the number of reps you do. Instead, concentrate on doing the exercise right and focus your mind on feeling the contraction of the muscle.

- *Maintain Tension*: To get the most out of every rep, you must not allow your muscles to rest at the top or bottom of a repetition. Try to maintain continuous tension throughout the entire range of motion.
- *Get a Peak Contraction*: For optimal results you need to hold the peak contraction for a second or two and really squeeze the muscle, then slowly bring it down.
- *Pull-up exercises* are extremely difficult. Some people I have trained cannot even do one repetition. If you fall into this category, try using a spotter. If you are working out by yourself, you can use negative resistance. Place a chair under the bar and begin in the up position, then lower yourself as slowly as possible. Negatives actually build strength more quickly than positive repetitions.
- I have provided *three different intensity levels* because everyone's strength in the beginning is different. Start with the lowest level for the first couple of workouts then move up to intermediate, when you feel that you are ready for more intense training.

Below you will find a training plan for beginners that raises the intensity levels incrementally. This is an excellent way to ease into a fitness program. Those of you who are not beginners can start with workout number four and progress from there.

Beginner Training Plan

Workout	# of Exercises	Sets per Exercise	Total Sets	Rest between Sets
(1)	5	2	10	2 minutes
(2)	5	3	15	2 minutes
(3)	5	4	20	1.5 minutes
(4)	5	5	25	1.5 minutes
(5)	5	5	25	1 minute
(6)	5	5	25	30 seconds

Upper Body			
Exercise	Beginner	Intermediate	Advanced
1	Low-intensity Push-up	Classic Push-up	Plyometric Push-up
2	Classic Push-up	Plyometric Push-up	Clap-in-the-Middle Push-up
3	Shoulder Press Push-up	Leg Lift Push-up	Rotational Push-up
4	Tricep Push-up	Tricep Push-up	Diamond Push-up
5	Low-intensity Pull-up	Curl Pull-up	Curl Pull-up

Lower Body			
Exercise	Beginner	Intermediate	Advanced
1	Jumping Jacks	Mountain Climbers	Mountain Climbers
2	Squats	Duck Squats	One-legged Squats
3	Alternating Lunges	Jump Squats	Jump Squats
4	Rope Skips	Calf Raises	One-legged Calf Raises
5	Crunch	Crossover Crunch	Bicycle

PEAK PERFORMANCE TRAINING

The primary objective of the *Hooked On Health* training system is to guide transformation aspirants to peak athletic performance, and by doing so, help them achieve the highest possible level of disease and injury prevention. The routines provided in this section will enable you to do just that — if you are ready for them. These workouts are extremely intense and have been written *only* for individuals who have been training with weights for a minimum of three months or who have completed the training sessions outlined in the preceding chapters.

The workouts in Chapter 13 are based on the principles of Bill Phillips' *Body-for-Life* program; however, you should know that these are not Phillips' exact recommendations. This is a convict's body-weight resistance training regimen inspired by Phillips and taught to me by Billy Dase, my transformation elicitor. With peak performance training we will combine resistance training, sprints for cardio and lots of yoga stretching in two completely different workout plans.

In Phase 3 you will use an upper-body/lower-body split that alternates on Monday, Wednesday and Friday. This split gives each body part three or four days' rest before the next training session, which, in my opinion, is optimal recovery time. These resistance-training workouts are designed to tax both the aerobic and anaerobic systems and are excellent for shedding fat. On Tuesday, Thursday and Saturday you will focus solely on sprints and stretching.

You will find some new concepts in these advanced routines. In Phase 3, your upper-body workout will include some cardio push-up pyramids. These exercises are difficult because they challenge your lactate threshold, cardio system and muscle fibers all at the same time. The Phase 3 lower-body workout is based on super-setting ab and leg exercises. While doing a set of one-legged squats, your partner will be doing ab work. Go back and forth without rest until you have completed four sets of each exercise, then rest for two minutes between super sets and get water. A total of four super sets gives you a grand total of 16 sets per body part. The pace of this routine gives you a good cardio workout, but one not as intense as the upper-body session.

After four weeks move on to Phase 4 to utilize a push/pull split, alternating on Monday, Wednesday and Friday, and a legs + cardio/abs + cardio split alternating on Tuesday, Thursday and Saturday. Here, the resistance training becomes even more intense, as specific muscle groups are isolated and overloaded. Each of these training sessions will take 45 minutes to one hour.

In Phase 4, we will utilize one of Phillips' strategies — a reverse pyramid with a compound super set. With the reverse pyramid you perform five sets of a given exercise and reduce the number of repetitions on each of the first four sets (12-10-8-6). Then, on your fifth set, you go back up to 12 repetitions, and immediately after your 12th rep, do a superset (also 12 reps) of a different exercise that targets the same muscle group but from a different angle. This method enables you to work the slow and fast twitch muscle fibers and cause an adaptation that develops endurance as well as strength and size. I have experimented with hundreds of different strategies and found that nothing works as well as this rep count. During the first four sets your muscles get comfortable as the lower reps match your fatigue level. Then when you go back up to 12, it shocks the fibers; and when you follow immediately with another 12 of a different exercise, you recruit fibers that you cannot hit any other way.

Another technique to use in Phases 3 and 4 is forced reps, which will require the assistance of a training partner. In fact, you cannot do these workouts without a partner. Forced reps are defined as performing an exercise to fatigue (failure) then pushing out more reps. For example, most individuals will not be able to make the 12-10-8-6-12-12 rep count on the pull exercises without assistance. If you fatigue on the eighth rep of the final set, your partner will help you get the last four reps by pushing you up over the bar. These repetitions can be insanely intense, but you will make your greatest gains if you can push through the pain and complete the specified number of repetitions.

With peak performance training your rest intervals between sets will be short — 30 to 60 seconds. Try to take only as much rest as necessary for your partner to complete their set; this pace keeps the workout moving and elevates your heart rate for some bonus cardio. You will still want to rest for a two-minute water break between exercises. In these phases you will also be training more frequently — six days per week — and that schedule will raise your metabolism even higher.

For a cardio workout nothing compares with sprints. Intense running (sprinting) is similar to doing squats in that it increases the release of growth hormone, which plays an important role in both muscle development and fat loss. It is also worth noting that with exercise, the more vigorous the activity, the lower your risk of heart disease. The heart is a muscle, and like other muscles in your body, will adapt to progressive overload and get stronger. Sprinting is also a perfect way to cultivate some lines of definition that your muscles cannot get any other way. Sprinting is an explosive form of strength training, and the more explosive muscle you build, the more fat your body can burn. Like the Olympic gymnast, sprinters' physiques — both male and female — are, in my opinion, the most beautiful, multifunctional on the planet.

With injury prevention in mind, you will ease into the sprinting regimen and spend more time warming up as well as stretching after the workout. In a four-week time frame you will do the sprint workout 12 times, three sessions per week. Following is an incremental plan that will quickly increase your cardiovascular strength:

Workout #1: (5) 50-yard sprints at 50 percent of your aerobic capacity (a brisk jog).
Workout #2: (6) 60-yard sprints at 60 percent of your aerobic capacity.
Workout #3: (7) 70-yard sprints at 70 percent of your aerobic capacity.
Workout #4: (8) 80-yard sprints at 80 percent of your aerobic capacity.
Workout #5: (9) 90-yard sprints at 90 percent of your aerobic capacity.
Workouts #6-#12: (10) 100-yard sprints as fast as you can possibly run.

Between sprints you should rest only as long as it takes to walk back to the starting point. You run a sprint, walk back, run a sprint, walk back. The workout does not take long, but is really intense. For the cool-down do five minutes of light jogging followed by five minutes of walking, then do the 20-minute yoga stretching routine.

Finally, your sprint workouts do not necessarily have to be running. You can apply the same training principles to swimming, cycling, stationary bike, kayaking, rowing, roller blading or even ice-skating. If you use any of these alternatives for your sprint training, use a watch to time your intervals: 50 yards equals 10 seconds, 100 yards equals 20 seconds, etc. My rest interval for a 100-yard sprint is 60 seconds (the time it takes me to walk back). Sometimes I will speed walk to cut the rest interval in half; this constitutes an active recovery phase that burns more calories. As your cardiovascular system gets stronger, work on speeding up the rest intervals. It is a lot tougher, but also produces better results.

Phase 3: Training Split

	Week 1	Week 2
Monday	Upper Body	Lower Body
Tuesday	Sprints & Stretching	Sprints & Stretching
Wednesday	Lower Body	Upper Body
Thursday	Sprints & Stretching	Sprints & Stretching
Friday	Upper Body	Lower Body
Saturday	Sprints & Stretching	Sprints & Stretching
Sunday	Off	Off

Upper Body		
Exercise	Sets	Repetitions
Warm-up		
Cardio Push-up Pyramid	5	$10^1 - 9^2 - 8^3 - 7^4 - 6^5$
Weighted Push-ups	5	$12 - 10 - 8 - 6 - 12$
Elevated Deep Stretch Push-up	5	$12 - 10 - 8 - 6 - 12$
Close Grip Pull-up	5	$12 - 10 - 8 - 6 - 12$
Double Triceps Extensions	5	$12 - 10 - 8 - 6 - 12$
Cardio Shoulder Push-up Pyramid	5	$5^1 - 4^2 - 3^3 - 2^4 - 1$ to failure
Cool Down		
On the pyramids 10^1 means 10 reps with 1 push-up, 9^2 means 9 reps with 2 push-ups, etc. Rest only 30 seconds or as long as it takes your partner to complete a set.		

Lower Body		
Exercise	Sets	Repetitions
Warm-up		
One-legged Squats	4	To Failure
One-legged Bridge	4	To Failure
2-minute rest between exercises		
Jump Squats	4	To Failure
Side Bridge	4	To Failure
2-minute rest between exercises		
Phantom Chair	4	To Failure
Crossover Crunch	4	To Failure
2-minute rest between exercises		
One-legged Calf Raises	4	To Failure
Plank	4	To Failure
Cool Down		

Phase 4: Training Split

	Week 1	Week 2
Monday	Push	Pull
Tuesday	Legs, Sprints & Stretching	Abs, Sprints & Stretching
Wednesday	Pull	Push
Thursday	Abs, Sprints & Stretching	Legs, Sprints & Stretching
Friday	Push	Pull
Saturday	Legs, Sprints & Stretching	Abs, Sprints & Stretching
Sunday	Off	Off

Abs, Sprints and Stretching				
Exercise	Sets	Repetitions	Compound Set	Repetitions
Warm-up Hanging Knee Raise	5	To Failure	Knee-up	To Failure
Hanging Leg Raise	5	To Failure	Reaching Crunch	To Failure
Oblique Knee Raise	5	To Failure	Opposite Arm & Leg Extensions	To Failure
Sprints	5 – 10			
Yoga Routine	20 min			

Push: Chest, Shoulders, Triceps				
Exercise	Sets	Repetitions	Compound Set	Repetitions
Warm-up				
Weighted Push-ups	5	12-10-8-6-12	Classic Push-up	12
Weighted Negative Push-ups	5	12-10-8-6-12	" "	12
Dips	5	12-10-8-6-12	" "	12
Shoulder Isolation Push-up	5	12-10-8-6-12	" "	12
Negative Double Triceps-Extensions	5	12-10-8-6-12	Triceps Isolation Push-up	12
Cool Down				

Pull: Back, Biceps				
Exercise	Sets	Repetitions	Compound Set	Repetitions
Warm-up				
Classic Pull-up	5	12-10-8-6-12	Low-intensity Pull-up*	12
Wide Grip Pull-up	5	12-10-8-6-12	Low-intensity Pull-up*	12
Horizontal Rows	5	12-10-8-6-12	Low-intensity Pull-up*	12
Bicep Isolation Curls	5	12-10-8-6-12	Low-intensity Pull-up*	12
Cool Down				

*You can raise the intensity substantially by doing the curl pull-ups instead of the low-intensity pull-ups.

Legs, Sprints & Stretching				
Exercise	Sets	Repetitions	Compound Set	Repetitions
Warm-up				
Weighted Squats	5	12-10-8-6-12	Jump Squats	12
Hamstring Curls	5	12-10-8-6-12	Jump Squats	12
One-Legged Calf Raises	5	12-10-8-6-12	Rope Skips	100
Sprints	5 – 10			
Yoga Routine	20 Mins.			

There will be times when your partner is not available and you must train alone. Following are some techniques I have used with consistent success when working out solo. Once you have completed Phases 3 and 4, consider working them into the routine you do with your training partner.

Reverse Gravity Isolation Principle is negative training taken to maximum intensity. Sometimes I like to do an entire workout that solely isolates negative resistance of a single exercise. On push, focus on dips, descending slowly (8 to 12 seconds) on the eccentric portion of the repetition, stop for a two-breath stretch at the bottom and then put your feet on the ground, allowing you to return to start without the positive repetition. You can do the same thing with the standard pull-up by putting a chair under the bar so that you can get up without the positive rep. Fifteen sets with 6–12 reps each of either exercise with 60-second rest intervals will make for a quick, efficient change-of-pace workout.

Partial Reps Training Principle is an excellent way to get forced reps without a partner. When you reach failure on a particular exercise

— pull-ups, for example — continue to pull yourself up as high as your strength will allow. The first rep beyond failure is usually 3/4 of a rep, the second a 1/2 rep and then probably a couple of 1/4 reps until your lats are fried.

Tri-Set Workout Principle is another quick, efficient way to work out by yourself. For example, begin with a set of deep-stretch push-ups, then immediately do a set of shoulder-press push-ups, and follow with a set of triceps push-ups. These energy-sapping sets require a 2-minute rest period. Usually, you can do 10 tri-sets in half an hour and tax all three muscles.

THE CONVICT'S LEAN AND MEAN WORKOUTS

In this chapter I will describe an advanced method of training that delivers simultaneous results in both muscle development and fat loss. The concept behind the Lean and Mean Workouts emerged slowly, strategically blending insights gained from reading *Muscle Media* magazine, John Hussman's thesis, *Why the Body-for-Life Program Works,* and the books *Sports Supplement Review,* by Bill Phillips and *Ultraprevention,* by Dr. Mark Liponis and Dr. Mark Hyman.

In the October 2001 issue of *Muscle Media* magazine, Senior Editor David Kennedy outlined the ultimate workout for cardiovascular fitness and fat burning, appropriately named Guerrilla Cardio. The regimen, originally developed by the Japanese National Speed Skating Team, is a high-intensity interval training system that intermixes eight intervals of 20-second maximum effort sprinting with 10-second rest periods between sprints. The entire workout takes only four minutes.

To test the effectiveness of this short but insanely intense regimen, Dr. Izumi Tabata of Japan's National Institute of Health and Nutrition compared it against a moderate-intensity cardio workout by measuring test subjects' VO_2 peak. Your VO_2 peak rates your cardiovascular system's efficiency in delivering oxygen to your working muscles. The bigger the number, the better your heart is at pumping blood to keep your muscles firing. In Dr. Izumi Tabata's study, the moderate intensity group rode an exercise bike for an hour a day, five days a week, at 70 percent of their VO_2 peak (the equivalent of jogging). The high-intensity interval training group rode on exercise bikes for four minutes of guerrilla cardio, five days a week, at 170 percent of their VO_2 peak (all out sprints). After six weeks, the moderate-intensity endurance training participants experienced a 10 percent increase in aerobic capacity and zero gains in anaerobic capacity. The guerrilla cardio group experienced a 14 percent increase in aerobic capacity and an extraordinary 28 percent increase in anaerobic capacity.[1] What makes this study so compelling is that other research demonstrates conclusively that when a person's anaerobic capacity increases, so does their metabolism and, subsequently, their ability to burn fat for 48 hours after the training session is completed.

Kennedy's article encouraged me to seek out more information which I found in Hyman's and Liponis' excellent book, *Ultraprevention*. The authors discuss the mechanics of why this type of training is so effective for fat burning. They state:

> **Interval training is a strong stimulus for our muscles to make more mitochondria; because when the heart and lungs can't produce any additional oxygen to the muscles, our muscles produce more mitochondria, in order to extract more oxygen from the bloodstream. There is a direct relationship between how much oxygen you breathe per minute and how many calories you can burn in that minute. If little oxygen is getting to your mitochondria, they'll burn calories very slowly.** [2]

Every individual has a different metabolic rate, like every different car has a different rate of energy efficiency, and the key to determining that rate is the mitochondria — the energizers within each cell that convert our food into energy (ATP). Having grasped this concept, I began to think about creating a workout to specifically train the mitochondria of every muscle cell in the body.

Not surprisingly, I found that professional bodybuilders had already invented one; a weight training method known as "drop sets." John Hussman's thesis, *Why the Body-for-Life Program Works,*[3] provided three important insights: (1) High-intensity resistance training is fueled by the ATP energy system; (2) maximum capacity for ATP is only 30 seconds for explosive force exercise; and (3) if you rest for 10 seconds the mitochondria can replenish the ATP energy stores. Professional bodybuilders drew on this science to develop the drop-sets method. For example, do a set of bench presses — 200 pounds, 12 reps. Then, rest for 10 seconds while your partner "drops" 20 pounds. Now do a set of 10 reps at 180 pounds. Next, rest for 10 seconds and your partner drops another 20 pounds. The procedure is repeated for three to eight drops, depending on your level of fitness.

Drop sets are the most advanced method of weight training for several reasons. First, the sheer volumes of sets expose your muscles to more overall time under tension. Second, the intensity is way off the charts. Third, you are actually exercising the mitochondria by forcing it to produce ATP at a greater rate. Fourth, and most importantly, from a health perspective, the sets strengthen the heart muscle.

Unfortunately, the California Department of Corrections does not provide weights for the inmates, so I improvised by creating a series of body-weight resistance training workouts that employ the principles upon which the drop-sets method was based. The Lean and Mean Workouts string together four consecutive body-weight exercises that target the same muscle group to form one "giant set." These exercises can be a more effective way to build muscle than drop-sets training, because four completely different exercises are used. Muscle fibers run in multiple directions; therefore, training a muscle from a variety of angles ensures stimulation of all its fibers for optimal growth.

In addition to being the most advanced method for developing muscle and shedding excess body fat, the Lean and Mean Workouts will dramatically reduce your risk of heart disease, the number-one cause of death in the United States. From research, I learned that elite endurance athletes have arteries that are 75 percent wider than normal, which reduces the risk of blockage that can lead to heart attacks and strokes. In order to widen your arteries (and strengthen the heart muscle), you need to increase the volume of blood that your heart is required to pump, exactly what these workouts are designed to do. This type of training will also enable you to develop a great cardiovascular infrastructure; not just in the heart and legs, but in every muscle in the body. Every part of your cardio system will perform at peak efficiency.

The following section details two completely different Lean and Mean Workout plans: The bulking phase for individuals who want to build huge muscles, and the cutting phase for those who want to focus on getting ripped.

Bulking Phase (5) Workouts

The bulking phase workouts are based on the following four new training principles that will challenge your muscles in ways in which they have never before been challenged.

Giant Sets: These sets consist of four consecutive body-weight resistance training exercises that tax the same muscle group from four completely different angles. This super-high-intensity set will enable you to tear the largest possible number of muscle fibers and also enables you to fully volumize the muscle. The key is to rest no more than 10 seconds between each exercise, so that before the blood leaves the muscle, you are already forcing blood back in. The body responds by creating new capillaries, which means more pathways for blood and nutrients to flow to muscle fibers.

Rest/Pause: The primary advantage of resting for 10 seconds between each of the four exercises is to replenish your energy stores. High-intensity resistance training is fueled by the ATP (adenosine triphosphate) and CP (creatine phosphate) energy systems. The max capacity for ATP and CP is about 10 to 30 seconds during explosive force exercise. Pausing for 10 seconds between exercises allows your muscles to recover rapidly by replenishing ATP and CP in muscles. As a result, rest/pause enables you to do a lot more volume, which leads to better results, because the muscle fibers are under tension for a much longer period of time.

Volumized Muscle Stretching: Upon completion of a giant set using the rest/pause principle, your muscles will be fully volumized, meaning that they are pumped to the max with blood containing glucose, creatine, amino acids and fluid. The muscle cells are surrounded by connective sheets, a girdle-like fascia with minimum elasticity. If you stretch a fully volumized muscle, you can "remodel" the girdle that confines your muscles, thereby expanding your capacity for growth.[4]

Double Sessions: A lot of professional bodybuilders work out twice a day to achieve optimal results. The primary benefit for the bulking phase relates to the intensity of your training. For example, by the time you complete a back workout, your biceps are quite tired. There is no way you can train them as hard as if you waited until later in the day and did a second session. With double sessions you need to do your first session in the morning, then wait at least six hours and consume three to four meals to replenish energy stores before the evening workout. You may even want to take a 20-minute afternoon or early-evening power nap to enhance recovery.

Bulking Phase Diet

If you want to develop extra-large muscles, then you need to consume more total calories and a lot of protein (1.5 grams per pound of body weight); for a 200-pound man this means about 5000 calories and 300 grams of protein every day. To attain this consumption without feeling bloated, I recommend that you drink several protein shakes. In a study conducted at Baylor University,[5] researchers discovered that consuming a mixture of whey and casein protein *before and after* resistance training increases muscle mass more than a single post-workout whey protein shake. Drinking an additional shake before your workout creates an ideal anabolic environment for muscle growth, as the additional amino acids can diminish the acute stress response associated with resistance training. You will still want to have a whole-food meal containing protein, a whole-grain carb and a fibrous vegetable about an hour after working out. Since you will be training twice a day, you will have a total of four whey protein shakes and two muscle-building, whole-food post-workout meals. For the rest of the day follow the basic guidelines set forth in the Connect with Nature Weight Loss Solution.

Bulking Phase Meal & Training Schedule

Time	Sample Meal Plan
6:20 a.m.	Blueberry-Citrus Smoothie (1 scoop of whey)
6:20–7:00 a.m.	AM Workout
7:00 a.m.	Strawberry-Banana Blast (2 scoops of whey)
8:00 a.m.	Spinach omelet*, whole-grain toast, glass of milk
10:30 a.m.	Peanut butter & honey sandwich on whole-grain bread
12:30 p.m.	Chicken breast, wild rice, asparagus spears
3:00 p.m.	Turkey sandwich on whole-grain bread
5:30 p.m.	Blueberry-Citrus Smoothie (1 scoop of whey)
5:30–6:00 p.m.	PM Workout
6:00 p.m.	Classic Whey Shake (2 scoops), 1 baked or sweet potato
7:00 p.m.	Salmon steak, whole-wheat pasta, salad
9:30 p.m.	Cottage cheese

*Note: Most bodybuilders eat egg whites because these are high in protein, low in calories and do not contain the cholesterol found in the yolks; you can buy them at EggwhitesInt.com. You may also consider two additional amino acid supplements: Carnitine, which has been found to increase testosterone receptor density, and Arginine, which causes the body to release nitric oxide. Nitric oxide increases blood flow and nutrient transfers to muscle tissues and promotes vascularity (bigger veins).

There are a number of different ways to split these training sessions depending on your schedule and your recovery needs. Here are four options to consider:

Bulking Phase Training Split

		2 on/1 off	3 on/1 off	4 on/1 off	5 on/2 off
Day 1	AM	Chest	Chest & Shoulders	Chest	Abs
	PM	Triceps	Triceps	Triceps	Chest
Day 2	AM	Legs	Legs	Quads	Abs
	PM	Abs	Abs	Hams & Calves	Back
Day 3	AM	Off	Back	Back	Abs
	PM		Biceps	Biceps	Shoulders
Day 4	AM	Back	Off	Shoulders	Abs
	PM	Biceps		Abs	Legs
Day 5	AM	Shoulders		Off	Abs
	PM	Abs			Arms
Day 6	AM	Off			Off
	PM				
Day 7	AM				Off
	PM				

I have experimented with all of these splits, and the simple truth is that they all work. For the most part, try to do a 40-minute workout for the larger muscles in the morning and a 20-to-30 minute session for the smaller muscles in the evening. Personally, I like the two-on, one-off because I like a lot of recovery days. Daniel, one of my training partners, prefers the five-on, two-off, because he likes to hit abs every morning before work and feels that his muscles respond best with six full days of rest per body part. Whatever split you choose, bear in mind that double-session resistance training workouts are extremely taxing on the body. I only train like this for two or three weeks at a time, then usually do a couple weeks of Walk in Nature Workouts before returning to the double sessions. If you start feeling rundown, take several days off. Daniel and I at times have both "burned ourselves out" with these bulking-phase workouts. After four or five days of rest, the body recovers and you come back stronger than ever.

Bulking-Phase 5 Workouts

Chest Giant Set	Shoulders Giant Set	Quads Giant Set
Dips	Handstand Push-up	Weighted Squats
Deep Stretch Push-up	Shoulder Isolation Push-up	Jump Squats
Classic Push-up	Upright Rows	Duck Squats
Negative Dips	Frontal Raises	Walking Lunges
Stretch Series #616	Stretch Series #617	Stretch Series #612

Triceps Giant Set	Biceps Giant Set	Back Giant Set
Double Triceps Extensions	Standing Curls	Wide-grip Pull-up
Push downs	Low-intensity Pull-up	Close-grip Pull-up
Triceps Isolation Push-up	Biceps Isolation Curls	Low-intensity Pull-up
Bench Dips	Neg. Biceps Isolation Curls	Pole Humpers
Stretch Series #618	Stretch Series #620	Stretch Series #619

Hams & Calves Giant Set	Abs	
Hamstring Curls	Pilates Series of Fives	
Calf Raises		
Neg. Hamstring Curls		
Neg. Calf Raises		
Stretch Series #613/#615		

Training Tips & Insights: Due to the intensity of these workouts you need to spend a little more time warming up. In addition to your regular warm-up you need to do one set of each exercise in the giant set.

- Rest 10 seconds between each exercise and two to five minutes between each giant set.
- Repetitions: Stop at one rep before failure on each exercise, usually in the 6-to-12 repetition range.
- The number of giant sets will be different for everyone and for each body part. The first time Daniel did the leg routine, he only did four giant sets and was sore for four days. It takes more sets to tear down the upper body. I normally do 6 – 7 for back, 9 – 12 for chest, 6 – 7 for shoulders, 7 – 9 for arms, 4 for hamstrings and calves and 5 for abs. You will have to experiment with different sets to determine what is right for your own body.
- Some new exercises in these workouts are essentially weight-lifting movements, which require one piece of equipment. In prison we just roll up a magazine for the handle and tie a rope (made from a piece of sheet) to it. Those of you in the real world can purchase a Flex Band which works great for these exercises.

- If you do not have a partner you will not be able to do the weighted squats. However, you can raise the intensity of squats without weight by going slowly — a five count on both the negative and positive portions of the exercise — and by holding the peak contraction at the top for a four count. On the final rep you can even hold the flexed position for 10 seconds.
- You may have noticed that there is no cardio mentioned here; that is because someone trying to bulk up needs to have a positive caloric balance. Cardio would simply burn up the calories you need to get big.

Cutting Phase (6)

In this section a two-week diet and exercise regimen is described that is specifically designed to push your metabolism to its highest point and accelerate your body's fat-burning potential. These workouts are similar to the bulking phase in that you will be using giant sets with the rest/pause principle for resistance training and be doing double sessions. The difference is that you will be doing resistance training in the AM session and guerrilla cardio during the PM session.

According to a study produced at the University of New Hampshire, you can burn more fat by splitting your cardio workouts into two separate sessions. Researchers divided 37 people into two groups; one exercised once daily for 30 minutes and the other did two separate 15-minute workouts. After 12 weeks, the group who did the double sessions increased their VO_2 max by nine percent and their total workout capacity by 21 percent — double the results achieved by the group who trained only once daily. Giant sets are essentially a cardio exercise, thus I believe that you can burn more fat with these workouts than with any other type of resistance training.

For the cutting phase you will be doing a shorter 30-minute giant-set resistance training workout in the morning and a quick guerrilla cardio and abs session in the evening. And just like Peak Performance Training you can do the sprints whatever way you prefer — running, swimming, cycling, stationary bike, kayaking or rowing.

Cutting Phase Meal and Training Schedule

Since your primary objective during the cutting phase is to burn fat, I'm going to recommend that you follow the Connect with Nature Weight Loss Solution with a couple of exceptions: (1) Drink your whey shakes with water; (2) eat veggies for your carbs in every meal with the sole exception of the post-workout, whole-food meals; this will cut about 300 calories out of your daily diet and raise your caloric deficit. With this workout and eating plan you will find the fat just melts off.

Mealtimes

Time	Sample Meal Plan
6:45 – 7:15 a.m.	AM Workout
7:15 a.m.	Whey shake with water, 1 banana
8:15 a.m.	Egg white omelet, oatmeal, select fruit
10:30 a.m.	Chicken breast, broccoli
1:30 p.m.	Salad with strips of turkey
4:30 p.m.	Tuna, tomatoes
5:30 – 6:00 p.m.	PM Workout (wait 1 hour before eating after cardio)
7:00 p.m.	Shrimp, whole-grain rice, mixed veggies

Cutting Phase (6) Training Split

	AM Session	PM Session
Day 1	Back	Guerrilla Cardio* & Pilates
Day 2	Chest & Shoulders	Guerrilla Cardio* & Pilates
Day 3	Legs	Guerrilla Cardio* & Pilates
Day 4	Arms	Guerrilla Cardio* & Pilates
Day 5	Off	Off

* Note: See David Kennedy's description of the Guerrilla Cardio workout on page 109.

Aerobic Training: Guerrilla Cardio & Pilates

Warm Up:	Jog for 5 minutes
	Stretch Series #612-615
	Pilates Series of Fives
Workout:	Guerrilla Cardio for 4 minutes
Cool Down:	Walk for 5 minutes
	Stretch Series #612-615
	Pilates Series of Fives

Note: This workout takes only 20 minutes

Cutting Phase (6) Giant Set Workouts

Back	Chest & Shoulders
Classic Pull-up	Dips
Static Hang	Deep Stretch Push-up
Low-intensity Pull-up	Shoulder Isolation Push-up
Pole Humpers	Classic Push-up
Arms	Legs
Standing Curls	Jump Squats
Push Downs	Duck Squats
Low-intensity Pull-up	Walking Lunges
Triceps Isolation Push-up	Calf Raises

Training Tips & Insights: These giant-set workouts are similar to those provided in the bulking phase, so the same basic principles apply with a few exceptions, as follows:

- With the exception of the back routine, these workouts are somewhat lower on the intensity scale because you will be training more muscles in one session, which leads to less volume.
- Rest 10 seconds between sets and only one minute between giant sets; this gives you some bonus cardio action and some extra caloric burn and gets it over with about 10 minutes faster.

Since everyone has a different level of strength, these exercises may be too difficult for some people and too easy for others. Thus, you are encouraged to experiment with different exercise combinations within the giant-set format.

Chapter

15

PAY IT FORWARD

In *Body-for-Life,* Bill Phillips summarizes his work by urging readers to guide someone else through his transformation program. He wants individuals who benefited from his book to share the wisdom with other people. He calls this sharing the Universal Law of Reciprocation, a concept that can literally change the world.

The title for Chapter 15 was inspired by one of my all-time favorite films, *Pay It Forward,* starring Kevin Spacey and Haley Joel Osment. In the movie, Spacey plays a teacher who assigns his students the difficult task of creating something that can change the world; to his surprise, one of them does just that. The character, played by Osment, proposes that if a person truly helps someone else transform their life, then asks the recipient to "pay it forward" by helping three other people turn their lives around, in time the number of individuals serving others will multiply exponentially, and it will change the world.

This extraordinary idea has made a profound impact on my own life, because when actually putting the principle into practice, magical things began to happen. As mentioned in Chapter 1, the *Body-for-Life* program in combination with Viktor Frankl's purpose in life therapy enabled me to overcome suicidal depression and discover a sense of purpose, in spite of the fact that I was serving a life sentence in prison. The changes I experienced were so incredible, I *had* to share them with someone else, so I paid it forward by guiding three other people — Charlie, Jim and Daniel — through the *Hooked On Health* program. Their stunning transformations inspired me to do something un-imaginable — write this book.

The pay it forward philosophy has also led to other exciting opportunities as I am now developing a venture called "The Youth Obesity Project." You may recall in Chapter 8 I discussed the creation of *The Amazing Weight Loss Formula* audio book, which combines Daniel Durland's tragic story of youth obesity with everything I have learned about losing weight (and that the audio book is available from my website as a free download). My hope is that readers of this book will pay it forward by telling all of their friends about the free audio download, and in so doing, help me help others lose weight. In the United States, 65 percent of the population is overweight. This statistic is so alarming that the Centers for Disease Control and Prevention recently announced that obesity is the most significant health issue of the 21st century; estimating that some 400,000 Americans die each year from health problems directly related to being overweight. My final piece of advice is this: Find three people who need help in this regard and guide them through the *Hooked On Health* program. I guarantee that it will be one of the most rewarding experiences of your life. If enough people follow Bill Phillips' example, "we" will indeed change the world.

One of the most amazing things about helping someone else without expecting anything in return is that the kindness comes back to you in unexpected ways. This principle is actually one of the basic constructs upon which the universe was built. According to Dr. Wayne Dyer, one of my greatest teachers, the purpose of the universe, of God, is to perpetuate life. And when our purposes are in sync with the purpose of the Universe, when we use our talents to serve others, our own life force, our health, becomes stronger.[1]

Over the last century a number of scientific discoveries have emerged to support Dyer's contention. One fascinating study found that a simple act of kindness toward another human being raised levels of the neuro-transmitter serotonin in the recipient, the giver, and even others who witnessed the act. High amounts of serotonin are associated with feelings of inner peace.[2] Human beings are genetically designed to provide value or service to one another. We are also designed with a specific purpose in life, "a concrete assignment that demands fulfillment."[3] I feel so strongly about this that I have written a second book titled, *Principles of Grace* that I hope will inspire others to discover the purpose of their own lives. This has become my personal mission and thus, I'd like to close with a preview of my next book.

Principles of Grace
A Sneak Preview

Principles of Grace proposes, through the medium of a parable, that the need for purpose is hardwired into every human being's soul and that this driving force is both instinctual and spiritual. The central theme of this book is that every human being is born with unique talents and passions, and when those natural abilities are expressed in a way that brings value or service to others, a direct channel to God's Universal Intelligence is opened. This opening results in a "receiving" of new insights, epiphanies and greater creativity.[1]

Abraham Maslow, one of the pioneers of modern psychology, devoted a lifetime to the study of individuals who achieved the highest levels of performance in fields such as sports, business, science and the arts. He described these peak performers as being self-actualized: "the process of discovering what it is you were born to do, and making a commitment to do it with excellence."[2]   Later he would revise his "needs hierarchy" theory and acknowledge that humanity's ultimate peak experience was not self-actualization but self-transcendence or living for a purpose higher than self.[3] Maslow's eternal wisdom has been echoed by some of the most profound thinkers of all time: Wayne Dyer, Deepak Chopra, Stephen Covey, Louise Hay, Viktor Frankl, Caroline Myss, Ralph Waldo Emerson, and Joseph Campbell, to name only a few. These enlightened souls teach that our universe functions on a principle of unity. Their message, which I hope to convey to the reader, is expressed most elegantly by Chopra in his *The Spontaneous Fulfillment of Desire:*

If you use your talents solely for the purpose of personal gratification, you will be out of sync with the universe. However, if you use your gifts to serve you and the larger purpose of unity, you will be in harmony with the universe and all of its resources will be made available to you.[4]

Principles of Grace is a parable (a short story that teaches a moral lesson). The book is designed to help readers discover and pursue their purpose in life. The story focuses on the lives of three characters— a sage of Native American descent, a middle school science teacher, and a troubled student—who draw on the teachings as each character faces various challenges and adversities.

The Principles of Grace are a collection of universal truths based on the culmination of ten years of research into peak human experience. The book condenses this wisdom into teachings that are passed down from one character to the next. In the section where the science teacher shares this knowledge with his troubled student, the lessons are displayed on 12 blackboards. This book is structured so readers can easily refer to the blackboard pages and apply the principles to their own lives.

In the process of compiling the Principles of Grace, I developed a passion for literature concerning human achievement and peak experience. I was particularly fascinated by the ground-breaking scientific discoveries that support spiritual principles. I learned that transcendent states of consciousness are available to us when our natural talents are dedicated to service. Through some mysterious force, noble intention activates our potential for greatness and empowers us to transcend perceived limitations. We begin to experience Divine inspiration—moments of grace.

Curiously, the research that I conducted to write *Principles of Grace* revealed time and again that sixth-sense experiences such as extra sensory perception (ESP), gut feelings, mothers' intuition, dream telepathy and clairvoyance are all related to something known as "unity consciousness." Thus, the 12 Principles of Grace that empower people to use their talents for the purpose of unity will also ignite their intuitive abilities.

The theory of unity consciousness has been around for thousands of years. The sage Pantanjeli wrote about the concept in the *Yoga Sutras,* which were published around 100 B.C. Consider Pantanjeli's insights regarding the potential associated with achieving unity consciousness:

> **When you are inspired by some great purpose all your thoughts break their bonds, your mind transcends limitation, your consciousness expands in every direction and you find yourself in a new, great and wonderful world. Dormant forces, faculties and talents come alive and you discover yourself to be a greater person by far than you ever dreamed yourself to be.**[5]

According to Wayne Dyer, the word "inspired" literally means to be *In Spirit*, to be one with spiritual consciousness.[6] When you are inspired or passionate about something, you gain access to higher intelligence—to the spiritual frequencies. When you focus that passion on serving the higher purpose of unity (i.e. serving others), your own consciousness connects with unity consciousness and miraculous things begin to happen. The Principles of Grace are about making conscious contact with this benevolent force and enabling it to work through you.

Principles of Grace empowers people to live a life in harmony with their deepest passions. The intuitive voice from within that says "I love dancing," or art or business or even raising children, is there for a reason.[7] When followed, that voice will lead to one's highest potential as a human being. Hopefully, this book will inspire readers to identify a noble purpose that resonates within their souls and also provide some tools to use on their transcendent journey.

THE ILLUSTRATIONS

Push Series
201 – Classic Push-up
202 – Low-intensity Push-up
203 – Wide Grip Push-up
204 – Diamond Push-up
205 – Leg-Lift Push-up
206 – Rotational Push-up
207 – Plyometric Push-up
208 – Clap-in-the-Middle Push-up
209 – Shoulder Isolation Push-up
210 – Handstand Push-up
211 – Triceps Isolation Push-up
212 – Double Triceps Extension
213 – Weighted Push-up
214 – Weighted Negative Push-up
215 – Elevated Deep Stretch Push-up
216 – Push Downs
217 – Dips
218 – Bench Dips
219 – Upright Rows
220 – Frontal Raises
221 – Cardio Push-up
222 – Cardio Shoulder Push-up

Pull Series
301 – Low-intensity Pull-up
302 – Static Hang
303 – Classic Pull-up
304 – Close Grip Pull-up
305 – Wide Grip Pull-up
306 – Curl Pull-up
307 – Standing Curls
308 – Horizontal Rows
309 – Biceps Isolation Curls
310 – Spotting Pull Exercises
311 – Pole Humpers

Leg Series
401 – Step Ups
402 – Walking Lunges
403 – One legged Calf Raises
404 – Calf raises
405 – Squats
406 – Duck Squats
407 – Weighted Squats
408 – One Legged Squat
409 – Phantom Chair
410 – Hamstring Curls
411 – Jump Squats
412 – Mountain Climbers
413 – Rope Skips

Core Training Series
501-505 Pilates Series
501 – Single Leg Stretch
502 – Double Leg Stretch
503 – Single Straight Leg Stretch
504 – Double Straight Leg Stretch
505 – Criss Cross Stretch-Bicycle
506 – One Legged Bridge
507 – Hanging Leg Raises
508 – Hanging Oblique Knee
     Raises
509 – Oblique Crunch
510 – Hanging Knee Raises
511 – Crossover Crunch
512 – Knee-up
513 – Reverse Crunch
514 – Plank
515 – Side Bridge
516 – Opposite Arm & Leg
     Extensions

THE ILLUSTRATIONS continued…

Yoga Stretching Series
Sun Salutation Series
601 – Prayer
602 – Mountain
603 – Forward Bend
604 – Lunge
605 – Plank
606 – Sphinx
607 – Cobra
608 – Downward Dog
609 – Lunge
610 – Forward Bend
611 – Mountain

Leg Series
612 – Quadriceps Stretch
613 – Hamstring Stretch
614 – Hips & Glutes Stretch
615 – Calf Stretch

Push Series
616 – Chest Stretch
617 – Shoulder Stretch
618 – Triceps Stretch

Pull Series
619 – Lat Stretch
620 – Biceps Stretch

Advanced Postures
621 – Shoulder Stand
622 – Spinal Twist
623 – Warrior

201-222 Push Series

201 Classic Push-up Targets: Primary: Chest, Shoulders Secondary: Triceps	
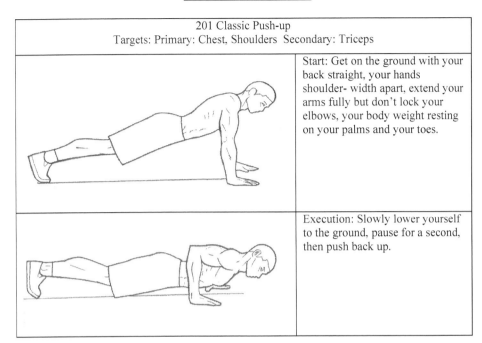	Start: Get on the ground with your back straight, your hands shoulder- width apart, extend your arms fully but don't lock your elbows, your body weight resting on your palms and your toes.
	Execution: Slowly lower yourself to the ground, pause for a second, then push back up.

202 Low-intensity Push-up Targets: Primary: Chest, Shoulders Secondary: Triceps	
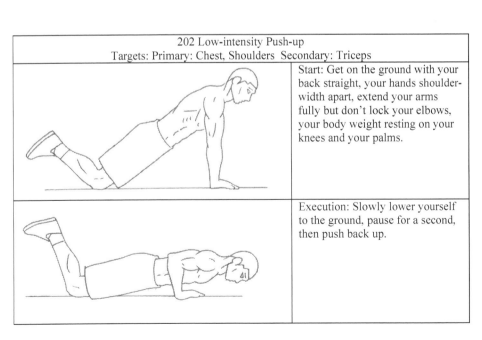	Start: Get on the ground with your back straight, your hands shoulder-width apart, extend your arms fully but don't lock your elbows, your body weight resting on your knees and your palms.
	Execution: Slowly lower yourself to the ground, pause for a second, then push back up.

203 Wide Grip Push-up
Targets: Primary: Chest, Shoulders Secondary: Triceps

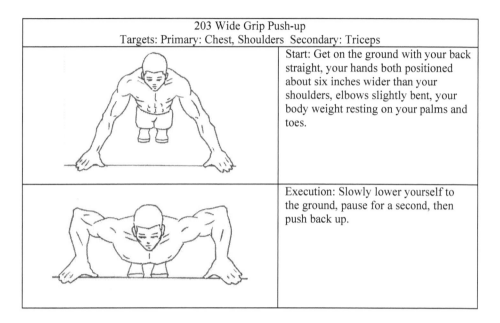

	Start: Get on the ground with your back straight, your hands both positioned about six inches wider than your shoulders, elbows slightly bent, your body weight resting on your palms and toes.
	Execution: Slowly lower yourself to the ground, pause for a second, then push back up.

204 Diamond Push-up
Targets: Primary: Triceps Secondary: Chest, Shoulders

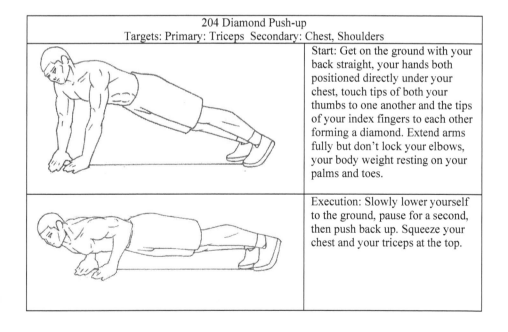

	Start: Get on the ground with your back straight, your hands both positioned directly under your chest, touch tips of both your thumbs to one another and the tips of your index fingers to each other forming a diamond. Extend arms fully but don't lock your elbows, your body weight resting on your palms and toes.
	Execution: Slowly lower yourself to the ground, pause for a second, then push back up. Squeeze your chest and your triceps at the top.

205 Leg Lift Push-up
Targets: Primary: Chest, Shoulders Secondary: Triceps

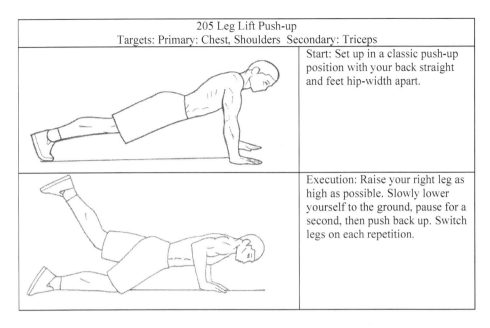

	Start: Set up in a classic push-up position with your back straight and feet hip-width apart.
	Execution: Raise your right leg as high as possible. Slowly lower yourself to the ground, pause for a second, then push back up. Switch legs on each repetition.

206 Rotational Push-up
Targets: Primary: Chest, Shoulders Secondary: Triceps

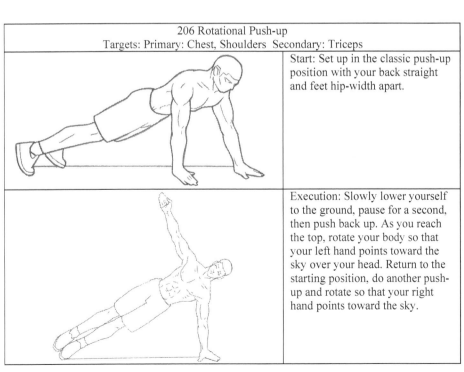

	Start: Set up in the classic push-up position with your back straight and feet hip-width apart.
	Execution: Slowly lower yourself to the ground, pause for a second, then push back up. As you reach the top, rotate your body so that your left hand points toward the sky over your head. Return to the starting position, do another push-up and rotate so that your right hand points toward the sky.

207 Plyometric Push-up
Targets: Primary: Chest Secondary: Shoulders, Triceps

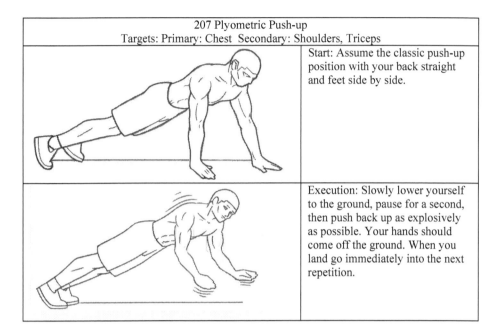

	Start: Assume the classic push-up position with your back straight and feet side by side.
	Execution: Slowly lower yourself to the ground, pause for a second, then push back up as explosively as possible. Your hands should come off the ground. When you land go immediately into the next repetition.

208 Clap-in-the-Middle Push-up
Targets: Primary: Chest Secondary: Shoulders, Triceps

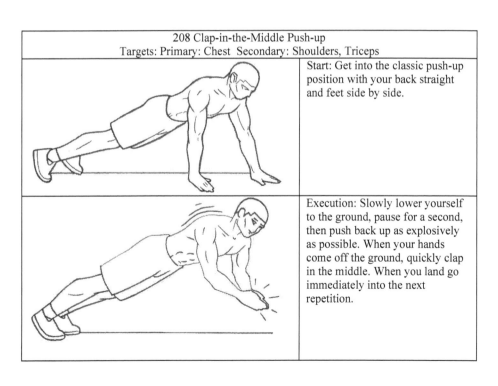

	Start: Get into the classic push-up position with your back straight and feet side by side.
	Execution: Slowly lower yourself to the ground, pause for a second, then push back up as explosively as possible. When your hands come off the ground, quickly clap in the middle. When you land go immediately into the next repetition.

209 Shoulder Isolation Push-up
Targets: Primary: Shoulders Secondary: Triceps

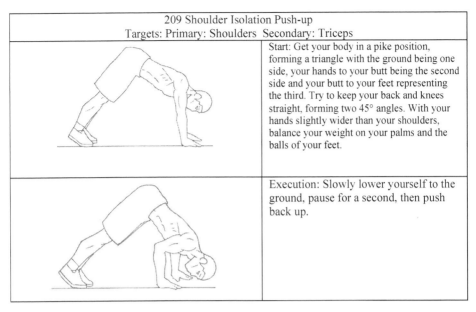

Start: Get your body in a pike position, forming a triangle with the ground being one side, your hands to your butt being the second side and your butt to your feet representing the third. Try to keep your back and knees straight, forming two 45° angles. With your hands slightly wider than your shoulders, balance your weight on your palms and the balls of your feet.

Execution: Slowly lower yourself to the ground, pause for a second, then push back up.

210 Handstand Push-up
Targets: Primary: Shoulders Secondary: Triceps

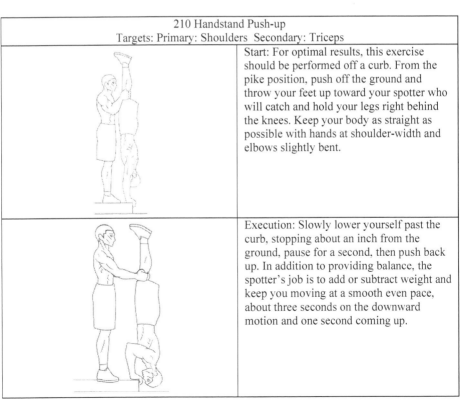

Start: For optimal results, this exercise should be performed off a curb. From the pike position, push off the ground and throw your feet up toward your spotter who will catch and hold your legs right behind the knees. Keep your body as straight as possible with hands at shoulder-width and elbows slightly bent.

Execution: Slowly lower yourself past the curb, stopping about an inch from the ground, pause for a second, then push back up. In addition to providing balance, the spotter's job is to add or subtract weight and keep you moving at a smooth even pace, about three seconds on the downward motion and one second coming up.

211 Triceps Isolation Push-up
Targets: Primary: Triceps

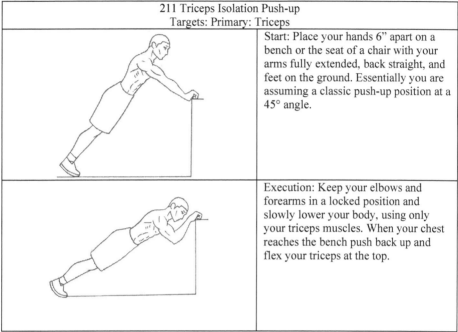

Start: Place your hands 6" apart on a bench or the seat of a chair with your arms fully extended, back straight, and feet on the ground. Essentially you are assuming a classic push-up position at a 45° angle.

Execution: Keep your elbows and forearms in a locked position and slowly lower your body, using only your triceps muscles. When your chest reaches the bench push back up and flex your triceps at the top.

212 Double Triceps Extension
Targets: Primary: Triceps

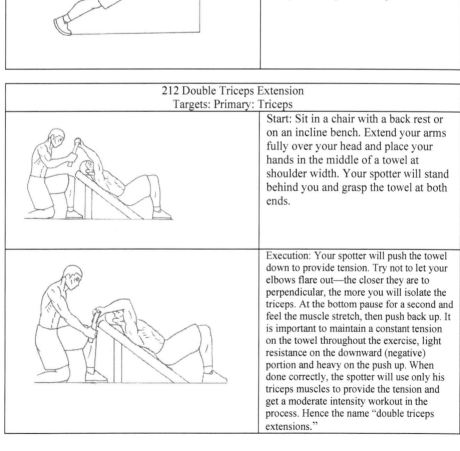

Start: Sit in a chair with a back rest or on an incline bench. Extend your arms fully over your head and place your hands in the middle of a towel at shoulder width. Your spotter will stand behind you and grasp the towel at both ends.

Execution: Your spotter will push the towel down to provide tension. Try not to let your elbows flare out—the closer they are to perpendicular, the more you will isolate the triceps. At the bottom pause for a second and feel the muscle stretch, then push back up. It is important to maintain a constant tension on the towel throughout the exercise, light resistance on the downward (negative) portion and heavy on the push up. When done correctly, the spotter will use only his triceps muscles to provide the tension and get a moderate intensity workout in the process. Hence the name "double triceps extensions."

213 Weighted Push-up
Targets: Primary: Chest, Shoulders Secondary: Triceps

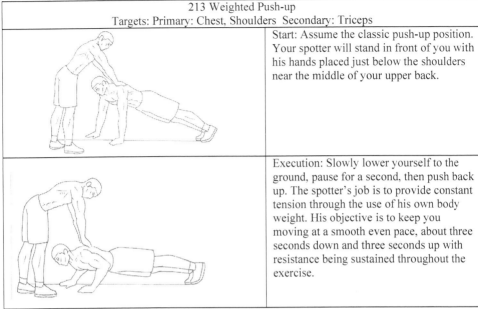

Start: Assume the classic push-up position. Your spotter will stand in front of you with his hands placed just below the shoulders near the middle of your upper back.

Execution: Slowly lower yourself to the ground, pause for a second, then push back up. The spotter's job is to provide constant tension through the use of his own body weight. His objective is to keep you moving at a smooth even pace, about three seconds down and three seconds up with resistance being sustained throughout the exercise.

14 Weighted Negative Push-up
Target: Primary: Chest, Shoulders Secondary: Triceps

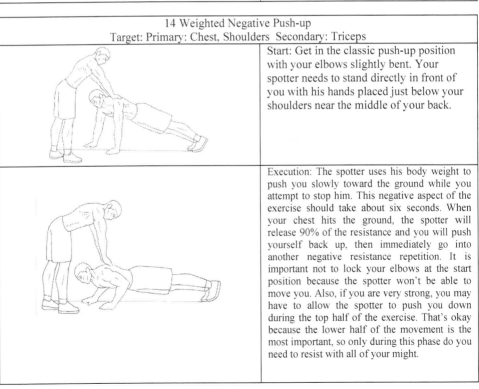

Start: Get in the classic push-up position with your elbows slightly bent. Your spotter needs to stand directly in front of you with his hands placed just below your shoulders near the middle of your back.

Execution: The spotter uses his body weight to push you slowly toward the ground while you attempt to stop him. This negative aspect of the exercise should take about six seconds. When your chest hits the ground, the spotter will release 90% of the resistance and you will push yourself back up, then immediately go into another negative resistance repetition. It is important not to lock your elbows at the start position because the spotter won't be able to move you. Also, if you are very strong, you may have to allow the spotter to push you down during the top half of the exercise. That's okay because the lower half of the movement is the most important, so only during this phase do you need to resist with all of your might.

215 Elevated Deep Stretch Push-up
Targets: Primary: Chest Secondary: Shoulders, Triceps

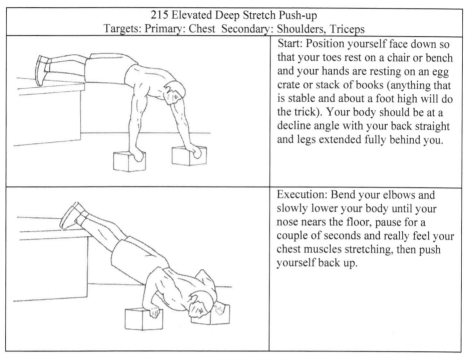

Start: Position yourself face down so that your toes rest on a chair or bench and your hands are resting on an egg crate or stack of books (anything that is stable and about a foot high will do the trick). Your body should be at a decline angle with your back straight and legs extended fully behind you.

Execution: Bend your elbows and slowly lower your body until your nose nears the floor, pause for a couple of seconds and really feel your chest muscles stretching, then push yourself back up.

216 Push Downs
Targets: Triceps

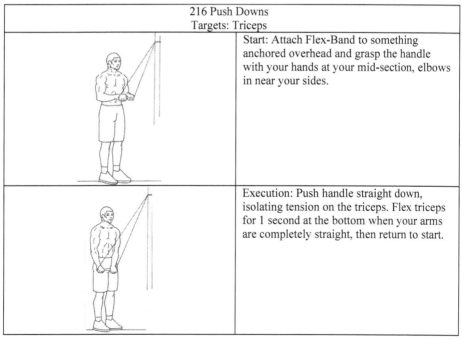

Start: Attach Flex-Band to something anchored overhead and grasp the handle with your hands at your mid-section, elbows in near your sides.

Execution: Push handle straight down, isolating tension on the triceps. Flex triceps for 1 second at the bottom when your arms are completely straight, then return to start.

217 Dips Targets: Primary: Chest, Triceps Secondary: Shoulders	
	Start: Grab a parallel dip bar with your arms fully extended and elbows slightly bent.
	Execution: Lean forward and allow your arms to flare out a bit as you slowly lower your body down, pause at the bottom for a second and feel the stretch on your chest, then push back up to start.

218 Bench Dips Targets: Triceps	
	Start: With your back to a chair, rest the palms of your hands on the seat with arms straight and fully extend your legs out in front of you at a 45° angle.
	Execution: Bend your elbows and slowly lower your butt toward the ground. You should feel tension on your triceps. Pause for a second at the bottom, then explode back up squeezing your triceps at the top of the movement.

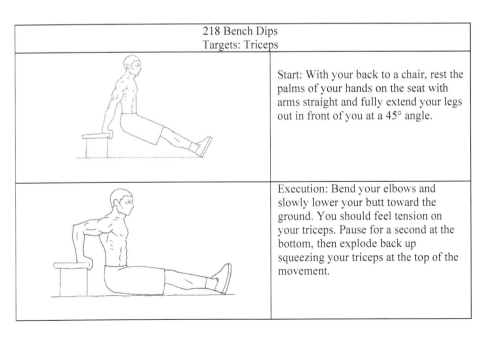

219 Upright Rows
Targets: Primary: Traps Secondary: Deltoids

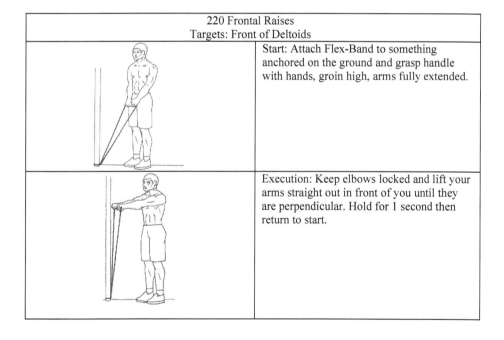

	Start: Attach Flex-Band to something anchored on the ground and grasp handle with hands, groin high, arms fully extended.
	Execution: Pull handle straight up to your breastbone, pause for a second to flex traps, then return to start.

220 Frontal Raises
Targets: Front of Deltoids

	Start: Attach Flex-Band to something anchored on the ground and grasp handle with hands, groin high, arms fully extended.
	Execution: Keep elbows locked and lift your arms straight out in front of you until they are perpendicular. Hold for 1 second then return to start.

221 Cardio Push-up
Targets: Primary: Chest, Shoulders, Cardio Secondary: Triceps

1 – Stand with your feet shoulder-width apart	2 – Quickly drop to a crouch so that your knees are touching your chest	3 – With your hands on the ground, shoot your legs to the rear so you're in the classic push-up position	4 – Do a push-up (or two or three)
5 – Draw your knees back to your chest	6 – Then quickly stand up again	7 – Do a jump squat.	Intensity Levels The basic cardio push-up is 1-7. You can increase the intensity by adding a second or third push-up or decrease it by eliminating the jump squat and adding a knee-raise and a toe-touch.
8 – Do a knee raise with your right leg	9 – Do a knee raise with your left leg	10 – Do a toe touch right hand to left toe	11 – Do a toe touch left hand to right toe

222 Cardio Shoulder Push-up
Targets: Primary: Shoulders, Cardio Secondary: Triceps

1 – Stand with your feet shoulder width apart	2 – Quickly move into a crouch so that your knees are touching your chest.	3 – Keep your hands on the ground and shoot your legs halfway back so you are in a pike position.
4 – Do a shoulder push-up (or 2 or 3, etc.)	5 – Draw your knees back to your chest	6 – Then quickly stand up again. That's one repetition.

301-311 Pull Series

301 Low-intensity Pull-up	
Targets: Primary: Back, Biceps	
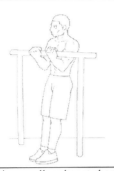	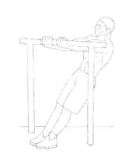
Start: Position a pull-up bar at chest level and grip it with your palms under the bar. Place your feet about six inches on the opposite side of the bar and rest your weight on your heels. Your body should be straight and at a slight angle.	Execution: Slowly lean back and extend your arms, with your feet remaining stationary, pause for two seconds and stretch your lat muscles, then use your biceps to curl yourself back to the start position.

302 Static Hang	
Targets: Primary: Back, Biceps	
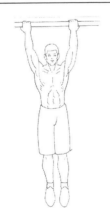	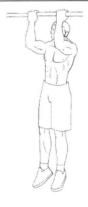
Start: Grab a chin up bar, using a shoulder width grip with your palms facing you, arms fully extended.	Execution: Pull yourself up a few inches to put tension on your biceps. Hold this position until your biceps begin to burn, then return to the start position and feel your back muscles stretch. Hold this position to failure.

303 Classic Pull-up Targets: Primary: Back Secondary: Biceps	
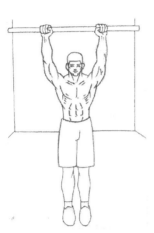	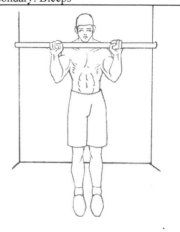
Start: Grab a chin up bar, using a shoulder width grip with your palms facing away from you.	Execution: Pull yourself up without swinging until your chin clears the bar, pause for a moment at the top before slowly lowering yourself back to start. Hang fully extended for a second to get a good stretch before doing another repetition.

304 Close Grip Pull-up Targets: Primary: Inner Back (rhomboids) Secondary: Biceps	
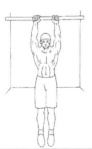	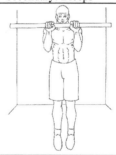
Start: Grab a chin up bar with your hands spaced about six inches apart and with your palms facing away from you.	Execution: Pull yourself up without swinging until your chin clears the bar, pause for a moment at the top before slowly lowering yourself back to start. Hang fully extended for a second to get a good stretch before doing another repetition.

305 Wide Grip Pull-up Targets: Primary: Outer Lats (wings)	
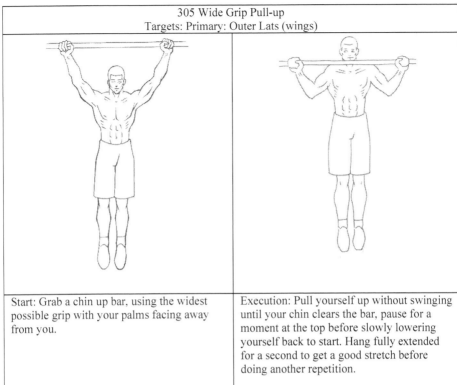	
Start: Grab a chin up bar, using the widest possible grip with your palms facing away from you.	Execution: Pull yourself up without swinging until your chin clears the bar, pause for a moment at the top before slowly lowering yourself back to start. Hang fully extended for a second to get a good stretch before doing another repetition.

306 Curl Pull-up Targets: Primary: Biceps, Inner Back	
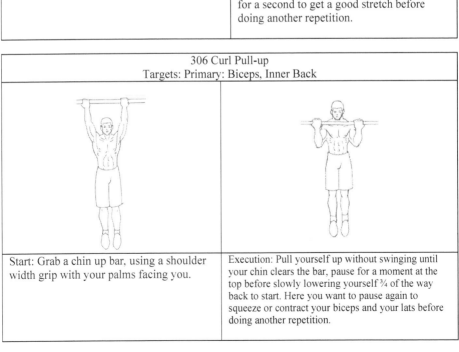	
Start: Grab a chin up bar, using a shoulder width grip with your palms facing you.	Execution: Pull yourself up without swinging until your chin clears the bar, pause for a moment at the top before slowly lowering yourself ¾ of the way back to start. Here you want to pause again to squeeze or contract your biceps and your lats before doing another repetition.

307 Standing Curls Targets: Biceps	
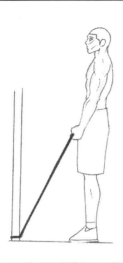	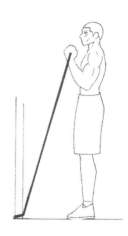
Start: Attach Flex-Band to something anchored to the ground and grasp handle, palms up about groin high with arms fully extended.	Execution: Keep your elbows at your sides and curl the handle up until your knuckles touch your chin. Flex your biceps for a 1 count and return to start.

308 Horizontal Rows Targets: Primary: Back Secondary: Biceps	
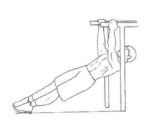	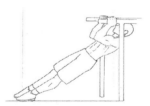
Start: Grab a dip bar with your knuckles facing the sky, your heels on the ground and your back straight. Your body should be at a 45 degree angle with arms fully extended.	Execution: Pull yourself up to the top, pause for a second then return to the starting position, pause for a two count and really feel your lats stretch before doing another repetition.

309 Biceps Isolation Curls
Targets: Primary: Biceps

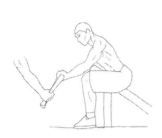 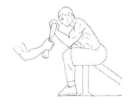

Start: Extend your arms fully over either a flat or incline bench and grab the middle of a towel or Flexband, whichever you prefer, with your hands six inches apart. Your partner will position himself on the other side of the bench and grasp the towel at both ends.

Execution: With your partner providing tension on the towel, slowly perform a curl, pause at the top then allow your spotter to pull you back to start. It is important to maintain constant tension on the towel throughout this exercise – heavy resistance through the (positive) curling phase and light resistance during the (negative) downward phase.

310 Spotting Pull Exercises

There are two different methods you can use to spot someone who is doing pull-ups. I prefer Technique A, but I encourage you to try both to see what works best for you and your partner.

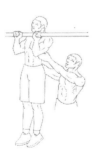 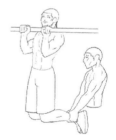

Technique A: The spotter places his hands on either side of his partner's back, just above the oblique muscles at the bottom of the rib cage and pushes straight up when help is needed.

Technique B: The person performing the exercise bends his or her knees at a 45° angle, and the spotter places his hands under their ankles. When assistance is needed the person performing the exercise may use leg strength to push up and/or the spotter can curl their weight in an upward direction.

311 Pole Humpers Targets: Lats	
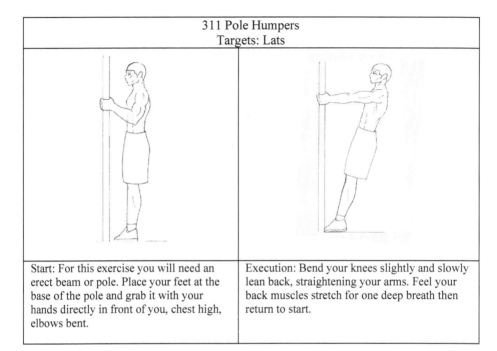	
Start: For this exercise you will need an erect beam or pole. Place your feet at the base of the pole and grab it with your hands directly in front of you, chest high, elbows bent.	Execution: Bend your knees slightly and slowly lean back, straightening your arms. Feel your back muscles stretch for one deep breath then return to start.

401-413 Leg Series

401 Step Ups Targets: Primary: Quads, Glutes Secondary: Hamstrings, Cardio	402 Walking Lunges Targets: Primary: Quads, Glutes Secondary: Hamstrings
Start: Stand with feet shoulder width apart in front of a step that's about a foot high. Execution: Step up with your right leg and then your left, then return to the start position. That's one repetition.	Start: Stand straight up with your feet together. Execution: Step straight out in front of you with your left leg and bend your right leg until your front thigh is parallel to the ground and the line from your ankle to your knee is perfectly straight. Pause, then step forward with your right leg and assume the start position. Repeat by leading with your right leg. That's one repetition.

403 One Legged Calf Raises Target: Primary: Calves	404 Calf Raises Target: Primary: Calves
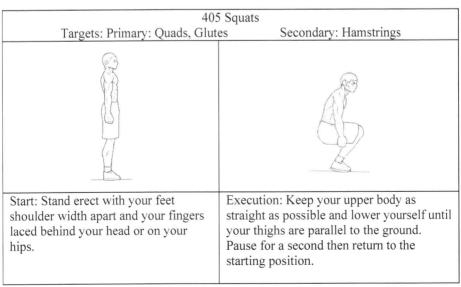	
Execution: Stand on one leg with the foot of your other leg resting on your heel to provide additional weight. Raise upward on the ball of your foot. Pause at the top and squeeze your calf as hard as possible, then return to the starting position.	Execution: Grab onto something for balance and slowly lift both of your heels upward. Pause at the top and squeeze your calves as hard as possible, then return to the starting position.

405 Squats Targets: Primary: Quads, Glutes Secondary: Hamstrings	
Start: Stand erect with your feet shoulder width apart and your fingers laced behind your head or on your hips.	Execution: Keep your upper body as straight as possible and lower yourself until your thighs are parallel to the ground. Pause for a second then return to the starting position.

406 Duck Squat	
Targets: Primary: Quads, Glutes	Secondary: Hamstrings
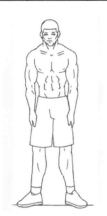	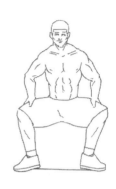
Start: Stand straight up with your feet farther than shoulder width apart and toes pointing out.	Execution: Keep your upper body as straight as possible and slowly lower yourself until your thighs are parallel to the ground. Pause for a second then return to start.

407 Weighted Squats	
Targets: Quads, Glutes	
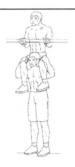	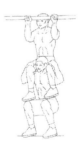
Start: Stand directly beneath a pull-up bar with your feet straight ahead and slightly wider than shoulder-width. Your training partner will then pull himself up and sit squarely on your shoulders. His feet should be at your mid-section and you can hold his ankles for balance. You can also put a board under your heels to emphasize the quads.	Execution: Inhale and hold your breath as you descend slowly, stopping when your thighs are parallel to the ground. Keeping your lungs full will increase the pressure inside your chest and abdomen to support your spine. Don't lean too far forward or allow your knees to pass over your toes. Return to start and exhale when you reach the top. Your partner, who is balancing his weight by holding the bar, can add or subtract weight as needed by pushing or pulling the bar.
Note: Do not attempt heavy squats if you have knee or lower back problems.	

408 One Legged Squat Targets: Primary: Hamstrings, Quads, Glutes Secondary: Calves	
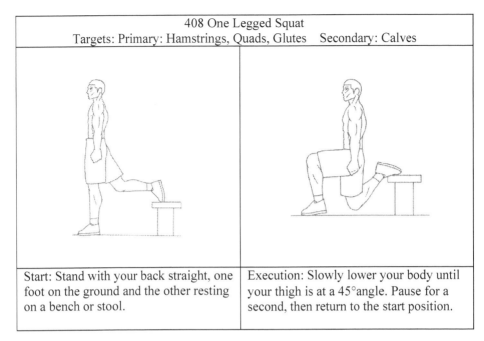	
Start: Stand with your back straight, one foot on the ground and the other resting on a bench or stool.	Execution: Slowly lower your body until your thigh is at a 45°angle. Pause for a second, then return to the start position.

409 Phantom Chair Targets: Primary: Glutes, Quads Secondary: Hamstrings	
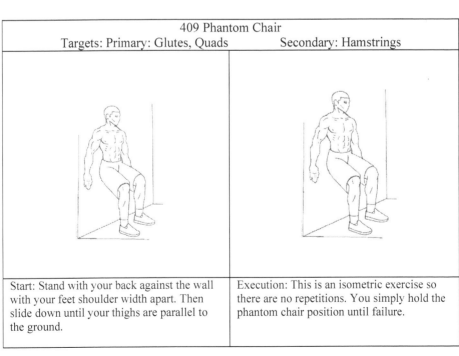	
Start: Stand with your back against the wall with your feet shoulder width apart. Then slide down until your thighs are parallel to the ground.	Execution: This is an isometric exercise so there are no repetitions. You simply hold the phantom chair position until failure.

410- Hamstring Curls Target: Primary: Hamstrings	
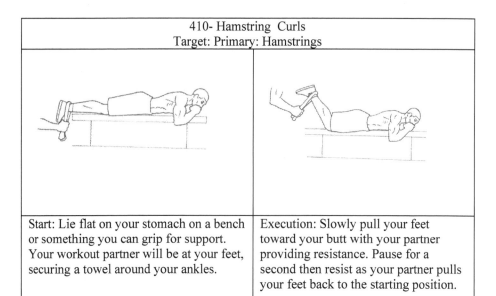	
Start: Lie flat on your stomach on a bench or something you can grip for support. Your workout partner will be at your feet, securing a towel around your ankles.	Execution: Slowly pull your feet toward your butt with your partner providing resistance. Pause for a second then resist as your partner pulls your feet back to the starting position.

411 Jump Squats Targets: Primary: Quads, Glutes, Hamstrings Secondary: Calves	
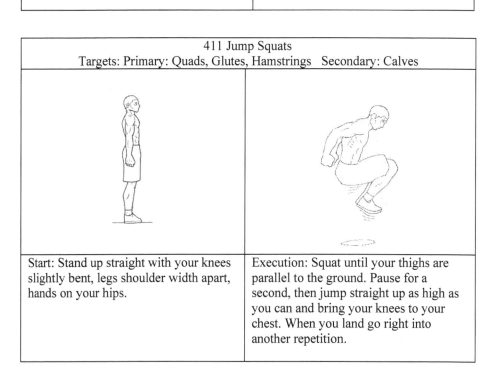	
Start: Stand up straight with your knees slightly bent, legs shoulder width apart, hands on your hips.	Execution: Squat until your thighs are parallel to the ground. Pause for a second, then jump straight up as high as you can and bring your knees to your chest. When you land go right into another repetition.

412 Mountain Climbers
Targets: Primary: Quads, Glutes, Cardio

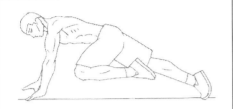 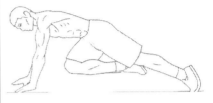

Start: Put your palms on the ground and assume the classic push-up position. Then pump your left leg.	Execution: Return to the start position, then pump your right leg forward. Repeat at a very fast pace.

413 Rope Skips	
Targets: Primary: Calves	Secondary: Thighs

Start: Stand up straight, feet shoulder width apart, knees unlocked, arms at your side holding a jump rope.	Execution: Swing the rope around your body front to back (or vise versa) and jump a couple of inches off the ground to allow the rope to pass under your feet. Land on the balls of your feet and immediately go into another repetition.

501 – 516 Core Training Series

501 Single Leg Stretch Targets: Primary: Abs Secondary: Hip Flexors	
Start: Lie flat on your back in a supine position.	Execution: Begin by hugging one knee to your chest while extending the other leg forward and resting it on the ground. Pause for two seconds to stretch the muscles. Switch legs on each breath.

502 Double Leg Stretch Targets: Primary: Abs Secondary: Hip Flexors	
Start: Hug both knees to your chest and feel your lower back muscles stretching.	Execution: Extend your legs forward slowly, keeping your heels together six inches off the ground, and simultaneously reach back behind your head with both arms in one flowing movement. Pause for a second then return to start. Hug both knees to your chest very slowly to stretch the lower back before doing another repetition.

503 Single Straight Leg Stretch
Targets: Primary: Abs Secondary: Hip Flexors, Hamstrings

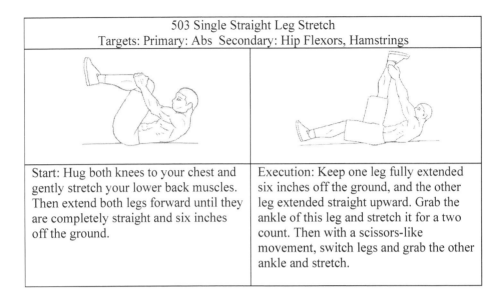

Start: Hug both knees to your chest and gently stretch your lower back muscles. Then extend both legs forward until they are completely straight and six inches off the ground.	Execution: Keep one leg fully extended six inches off the ground, and the other leg extended straight upward. Grab the ankle of this leg and stretch it for a two count. Then with a scissors-like movement, switch legs and grab the other ankle and stretch.

504 Double Straight Leg Stretch
Targets: Primary: Lower Back Secondary: Abs

Start: Lie flat on your stomach with arms and legs fully extended.	Execution: Without bending the elbows or knees, simultaneously lift your arms and legs six inches off the ground. Hold for one second and feel your lower back muscles contract, then return to lying flat on the ground.

NOTE: 501-505 is the Pilates Series. When performing the Pilates Series of Fives, you do all five exercises, one after the other, without resting between exercises.

505 Criss-Cross Stretch (Bicycle) Targets: Primary: Abs

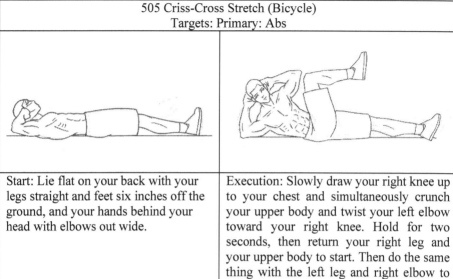

Start: Lie flat on your back with your legs straight and feet six inches off the ground, and your hands behind your head with elbows out wide.	Execution: Slowly draw your right knee up to your chest and simultaneously crunch your upper body and twist your left elbow toward your right knee. Hold for two seconds, then return your right leg and your upper body to start. Then do the same thing with the left leg and right elbow to complete one repetition.

506 One Legged Bridge Targets: Primary: Lower Back

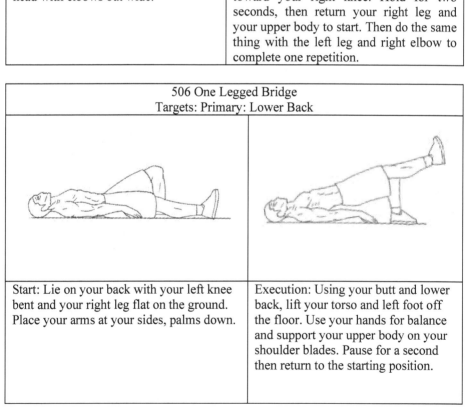

Start: Lie on your back with your left knee bent and your right leg flat on the ground. Place your arms at your sides, palms down.	Execution: Using your butt and lower back, lift your torso and left foot off the floor. Use your hands for balance and support your upper body on your shoulder blades. Pause for a second then return to the starting position.

507 Hanging Leg Raises
Targets: Primary: Abs   Secondary: Back

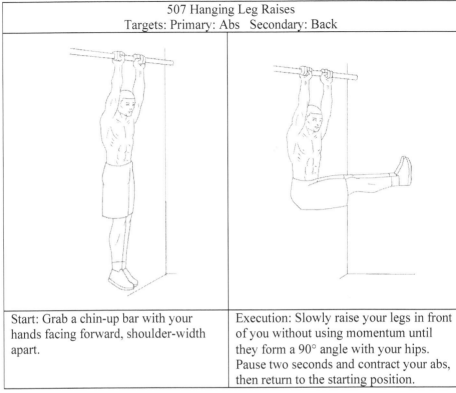

Start: Grab a chin-up bar with your hands facing forward, shoulder-width apart.

Execution: Slowly raise your legs in front of you without using momentum until they form a 90° angle with your hips. Pause two seconds and contract your abs, then return to the starting position.

508 Hanging Oblique Knee Raises
Targets: Primary: Obliques   Secondary: Abs, Back, Serratus

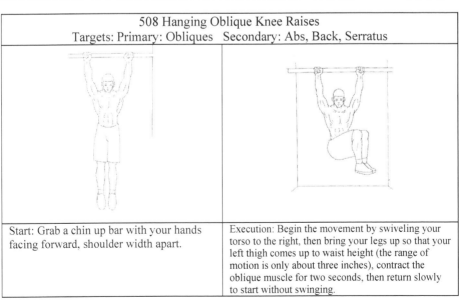

Start: Grab a chin up bar with your hands facing forward, shoulder width apart.

Execution: Begin the movement by swiveling your torso to the right, then bring your legs up so that your left thigh comes up to waist height (the range of motion is only about three inches), contract the oblique muscle for two seconds, then return slowly to start without swinging.

509 Oblique Crunch
Targets: Primary: Obliques, Serratus   Secondary: Abs

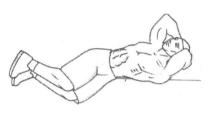 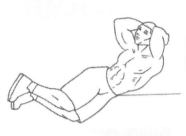

Start: Lie on the floor and allow your knees and hips to roll over to one side. Try to keep your shoulders square to the ground so that you are looking straight toward the sky, with your hands behind your head, elbows flared out.	Execution: Keep your shoulders square to the ground and crunch your upper body straight up toward the sky, contracting your oblique muscles. Pause for a two count, then return to the starting position. Rep out to failure, then switch sides.

510 Hanging Knee Raises
Targets: Primary: Abs Secondary: Back

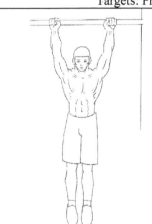 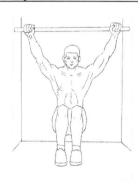

Start: Grab a chin up bar with both hands facing forward, shoulder width apart. Keep your back straight and your feet together.	Execution: Slowly raise your knees to waist height without swinging your legs, pause two seconds and contract your abs as hard as you can, then return to the starting position.

511 Crossover Crunch Targets: Primary: Abs Secondary: Serratus, Obliques	
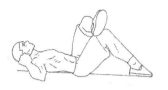	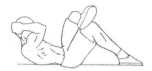
Start: Lie flat on the ground with your right leg bent, knee pointing toward the sky and your foot flat on the ground. Then sit your left ankle on top of your right knee. Place your fingers behind your head, with elbows flared out.	Execution: Lift your shoulders and upper body off the ground by contracting your abs, then twist your torso and touch right elbow to your left knee. Pause for a two count, then slowly lower back down. When you reach the ground immediately transition back into another repetition. By not stopping you will maintain constant tension on the target muscle group.

512 Knee-up Targets: Primary: Abs Secondary: Hip Flexors	
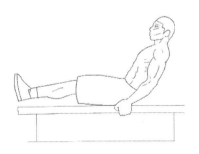	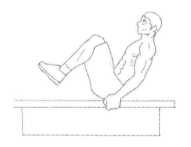
Start: Position yourself at the end of a bench and grip the sides of it behind your back. Lean back with your upper torso and extend your legs off the bench with a bend in your knees, balancing your body weight on your butt.	Execution: Moving only your legs, bring your knees toward your chest and contract your abs. Pause for a second, then push your feet back to the starting position.

513 Reverse Crunch Targets: Primary: Abs Secondary: Hip Flexors	
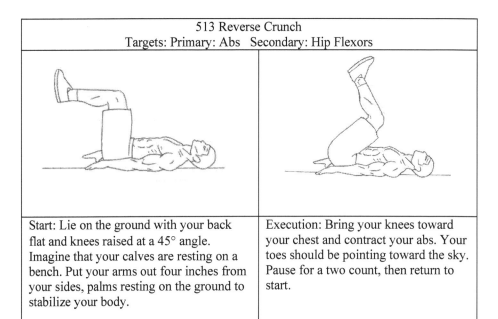	
Start: Lie on the ground with your back flat and knees raised at a 45° angle. Imagine that your calves are resting on a bench. Put your arms out four inches from your sides, palms resting on the ground to stabilize your body.	Execution: Bring your knees toward your chest and contract your abs. Your toes should be pointing toward the sky. Pause for a two count, then return to start.

514 Plank Targets: Primary: Abs	
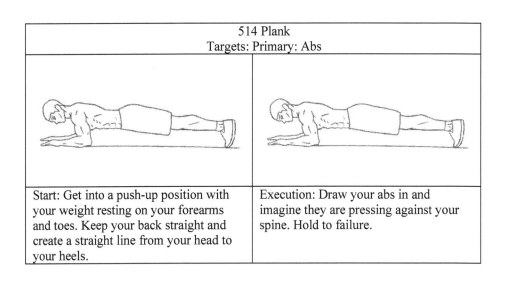	
Start: Get into a push-up position with your weight resting on your forearms and toes. Keep your back straight and create a straight line from your head to your heels.	Execution: Draw your abs in and imagine they are pressing against your spine. Hold to failure.

515 Side Bridge Targets: Primary: Obliques Secondary: Abs	
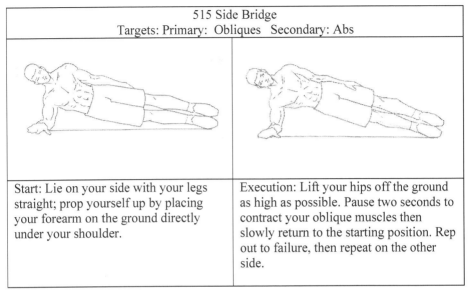	
Start: Lie on your side with your legs straight; prop yourself up by placing your forearm on the ground directly under your shoulder.	Execution: Lift your hips off the ground as high as possible. Pause two seconds to contract your oblique muscles then slowly return to the starting position. Rep out to failure, then repeat on the other side.

516 Opposite Arm & Leg Extension Targets: Primary: Lower Back	
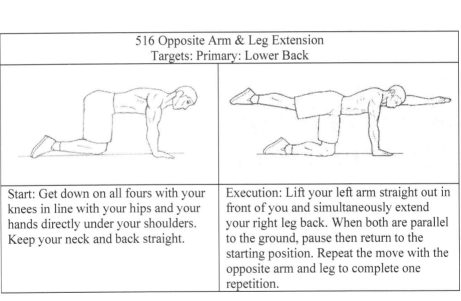	
Start: Get down on all fours with your knees in line with your hips and your hands directly under your shoulders. Keep your neck and back straight.	Execution: Lift your left arm straight out in front of you and simultaneously extend your right leg back. When both are parallel to the ground, pause then return to the starting position. Repeat the move with the opposite arm and leg to complete one repetition.

601-623 Yoga Stretching Series

Sun Salutation 601 - 611			
601 – Prayer – Begin by standing with your feet together and palms together in front of your chest prayer style. Take 3 deep breaths.	602 – Mountain – Inhale and raise both of your arms up, fingers pointing toward the sky and out slightly, forming a V.	603 – Forward Bend – Exhale and bend forward bringing your belly and chest toward thighs and hands to your feet.	604 – Lunge – Inhale and bring your right foot all the way back, your chest touching your left thigh and arms parallel with the right calf.
605 – Plank – Exhale and bring right foot back alongside the left, hands on ground, arms straight — like the up position of the classic push-up.	606 – Sphinx – Inhale and slowly lower your body to just a couple inches off the ground — like the down position of the classic push-up.	607 – Cobra – Exhale and push your chest up, straighten your arms while leaving the lower half of your body just a few inches off the ground.	608 – Downward Dog – Inhale and take a small step forward with both feet, leaving hands flat on the ground, and raise your butt toward the sky, forming two 45° angles. Rest for one deep breath.
			Trainer's Note: The Sun Salutation is a flowing series of poses that change with each breath. Inhale when the body opens and exhale when it closes. Repeat series a minimum of 4 times.
609 – Lunge – Inhale and slowly move into the lunge position; however, this time bring your right leg forward.	610 – Forward Bend – Exhale and bring your left leg forward transitioning to the forward bend position.	611 – Mountain – Inhale and raise both of your arms up, fingers pointing toward the sky.	

612 – Quadriceps Stretch	613– Hamstring Stretch
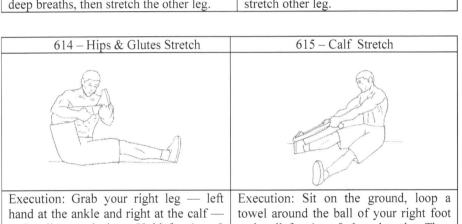	
Execution: Bend your right knee, bringing your heel up to buttocks. Grasp ankle with right hand and stretch. Hold for 4 or 8 deep breaths, then stretch the other leg.	Execution: Bend your torso forward and grab your left leg with both hands. Hold for 4 or 8 deep breaths, then stretch other leg.

614 – Hips & Glutes Stretch	615 – Calf Stretch
Execution: Grab your right leg — left hand at the ankle and right at the calf — and pull toward chest. Hold for 4 or 8 deep breaths, then stretch the other leg.	Execution: Sit on the ground, loop a towel around the ball of your right foot and pull for 4 or 8 deep breaths. Then stretch the other calf.

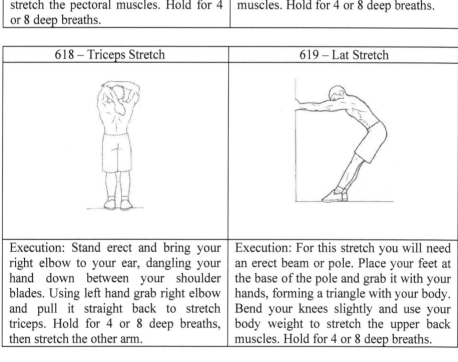

616 – Chest Stretch	617 – Shoulder Stretch
Execution: Use an open doorway, placing your arms on the wall on either side of the opening. Lean your body weight evenly through the opening to stretch the pectoral muscles. Hold for 4 or 8 deep breaths.	Execution: Use an open doorway or a pull-up bar, and grasp it with arms fully extended overhead. Then lean your bodyweight forward to stretch shoulder muscles. Hold for 4 or 8 deep breaths.

618 – Triceps Stretch	619 – Lat Stretch
Execution: Stand erect and bring your right elbow to your ear, dangling your hand down between your shoulder blades. Using left hand grab right elbow and pull it straight back to stretch triceps. Hold for 4 or 8 deep breaths, then stretch the other arm.	Execution: For this stretch you will need an erect beam or pole. Place your feet at the base of the pole and grab it with your hands, forming a triangle with your body. Bend your knees slightly and use your body weight to stretch the upper back muscles. Hold for 4 or 8 deep breaths.

620 – Biceps Stretch	621 – Shoulder Stand
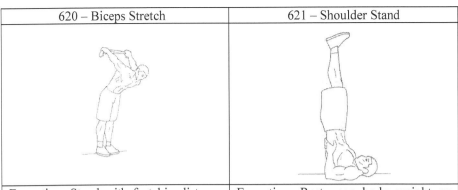	
Execution: Stand with feet hip distance apart, hold a towel/strap in both hands behind body. Bending slightly forward, lift arms while pulling outward until you find the resistance on the front of the arm. Hold for 4 or 8 deep breaths. Relax arms and return to starting position. Repeat 3 times.	Execution: Rest your body weight on your shoulders and triceps, which should be flat on the ground. Place your hands on your lower back. Extend your legs straight up with toes facing the sky, and balance weight on the shoulders and triceps. Hold the position for 4 or 8 deep breaths.

622 – Spinal Twist	623 - Warrior
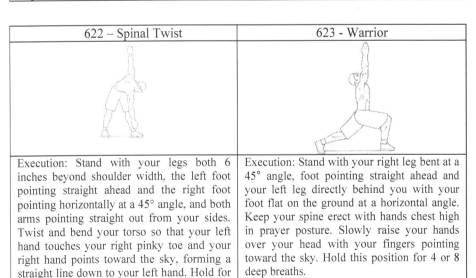	
Execution: Stand with your legs both 6 inches beyond shoulder width, the left foot pointing straight ahead and the right foot pointing horizontally at a 45° angle, and both arms pointing straight out from your sides. Twist and bend your torso so that your left hand touches your right pinky toe and your right hand points toward the sky, forming a straight line down to your left hand. Hold for 4 or 8 deep breaths.	Execution: Stand with your right leg bent at a 45° angle, foot pointing straight ahead and your left leg directly behind you with your foot flat on the ground at a horizontal angle. Keep your spine erect with hands chest high in prayer posture. Slowly raise your hands over your head with your fingers pointing toward the sky. Hold this position for 4 or 8 deep breaths.

End Notes

Chapter 1: Hooked On Health

1 Frankl, V.E., *Man's Search for Meaning: An Introduction to Logotherapy.* Buckaneer Books. 1993.
2 Ibid.
3 Covey, S.R., *The 7 Habits of Highly Effective People: Powerful Lessons in Personal Change.* Simon and Schuster. 1990.
4 Pine, B.J. and J.H. Gilmore, *The Experience Economy.* Harvard Business School Press. 1999.
5 Phillips, B., *Body-for-Life.* Harper Collins. 1999.
6 Lemonick, M.D., "Your Mind, Your Body." *Time.* Jan. 30, 2003.
7 Hyman, M. and M. Liponis, *Ultraprevention.* Scribner. 2003.
8 Antonio, J. and J. Stout., *Sports Supplements.* Lippincott, Williams and Wilkins. 2001. (p. 19-22)
9 Hyman, M., *Ultrametabolism.* Scribner. 2006. (p. 17)
10 Whitmarsh, B., *Mind and Muscle.* Human Kinetics. 2001.

Chapter 2: Medical Science's 20 Fat Loss Secrets

1 National Center for Health Statistics, Centers for Disease Control. "Prevalence of Overweight and Obesity Among Adults: United States, 1999." HTTP://CDC.gov/NCHA/products/pulis/pupd/hestats/obese/obese99.htm Accessed 9/5/2001
2 Mokdad, A.H., "Actual causes of death in the United States, 2000." *JAMA.* 2004. 291: 1238-1245.
3 Helmich, N., "Extra weight shaves years off your life." *USA Today.* Jan. 7, 2003.
4 "Second study finds obesity shortens life." *USA Today.* Jan. 14, 2003.
5 Blechman, S. and Steve Fahey, "Research-Fat Loss." *Muscular Development.* Volume 45, Number 8, August 2008 (p. 94)
6 Samara, J.N., "Patterns and trends in food portion sizes," 1997-1998. *JAMA.* 2003. 289: 450-453.
7 Phillips, B., *Sports Supplement Review.* Mile High Publishing. 1999. (p. 264)
8 Jenkins, D.J. et al., "Nibbling versus Gorging: Metabolic advantages of increased meal frequency." *NEJM.* 1989. 321 (14): 929-934.
9 Hussman, J., "Why the Body-for-Life Program Works." http//www.hussman.com/EAS Accessed 1/21/01
10 Stoppani, J., "Spot On Supps: Go the extra mile in your quest for the ripped six pack you've always wanted with these five scientifically proven fat burning supplements." *Muscle & Fitness.* 2007. 68(6): 153
11 Nobels, F., et al., "Weight Reduction with a High Protein, Low Carbohydrate, Calorie Restricted Diet: Effects on Blood Pressure, Glucose and Insulin Levels." *Netherlands Journal of Medicine,* 35 (5-6). 1989. 259-302.

12 Mourier, A. et al., "Combined effects of calorie restriction and branch-chain amino acid supplementation on body composition and exercise performance in elite wrestlers." *International Journal of Sports Medicine.* 1997. 18: 47-55.

13 Bell, E.A. and B.J. Rolls, "Energy density of foods effect energy intake across multiple levels of fat content in lean and obese women." *American Journal of Clinical Nutrition.* 2001. 73(6): 1010-1018.

14 Wyatt, H.R., "Long term weight loss and breakfast in subjects in the National Weight Control Registry." *Obesity Res.* 2002. Feb; 10(2): 78-82.

15 Aceto, C. and E. Velazquez, "Never Diet Again: Do away with dieting altogether by incorporating these 12 simple adjustments into your everyday nutrition and training programs." *Muscle & Fitness.* 2007. 68(5): 184-192.

16 Perricone, N. *The Perricone Weight Loss Diet.* Ballantine Books, 2005. (p. 49-50)

17 Alexander, C., "Fat Loss Handbook, Cause for Concern #2 The Boob Toob." *Men's Fitness.* 2003. Feb. (p. 85)

18 Chandalia, M., "Beneficial Effects of High Fiber intake in patients with Type 2 Diabetes Mellitus." *NEJM.* 342, 2000. (p. 1392-1398)

19 Chopra, Deepak and D. Simon, *Training the Mind — Healing the Body.* (Audio series) Nightingale-Conant. 1997.

Chapter 3: Aerobic Training

1 www.howstuffworks.com, "How Metabolism Works"

2 Hyman, M., *Ultrametabolism.* Scribner. 2006. (p. 156)

3 Ibid. (p. 161)

4. Tremblay, A. et al., "Impact of exercise intensity on body fatness and skeletal muscle metabolism." *Metabolism.* 1994 Jul; 43(7): 814-818

5 Chopra, D. and D. Simon, *Training the Mind, Healing the Body.* (Audio series) Nightingale-Conant. 1997.

Chapter 4: Resistance Training

1 Hyman, M., *Ultrametabolism.* Scribner. 2006. (p. 17)

2 Romano, J. "The Way I See It — The Romano Factor." *Muscular Development.* Volume 45, Number 8. August 2008. (p. 56)

3 Hussman, J., "Why the *Body-for-Life* Program Works." http//www.hussman.com/EAS/p3. Accessed 1/21/01.

4 Ibid. (p. 5)

5 Phillips, B. *Sports Supplement Review.* Mile High Publishing. 1999.

6 Whitmarsh, B., *Mind and Muscle: Psyche Up, Build Up.* Human Kinetics. 2001.

7 Ibid.

8 Ibid.

9 Ibid.

10 Ibid.

11 Hussman, J., "Why the *Body-for-Life* Program Works." http//www.hussman.com/EAS/p7. Accessed 1/21/01.

12 Ibid. (p. 8)

Chapter 5: Rest and Recovery

1 Stoppani, J. and J. Wuebben, "Tuning into the Right Frequency." *Muscle & Fitness.* 2007; 68(5) 210-222.

2 Gangwisch, J. et al., Columbia University Mailman School of Public Health and the Obesity Research Center Study, 2004.

3 Moore, P., "Good Night and Good Luck." *Men's Health.* 2006. December. pp. 151-159.

4 Chopra, D. and D. Simon, *Training the Mind, Healing the Body.* (Audio series) Nightingale-Conant. 1997.

5 Devereau, G., *Dynamic Yoga: The Ultimate Workout That Chills Your Mind As It Changes Your Body.* Thorsons GBR. 1999.

6 Pan, W.J. and A.R. Johnson, et al., "Reduction of chemical sensitivity by means of heat depuration, physical therapy and nutritional supplementation in a controlled environment." *J Nutr Env Med.* 1996; 6: 141-148.

7 Pelletier, C. et al., "Energy balance and pollution by organochlorines and polychlorinated biphenyls." *Obesity Review.* 2003 Feb.; 4(1): 17-24. Review.

Chapter 6: Proper Nutrition

1 www.howstuffworks.com, "How Metabolism Works"

2 Hussman, J., "Why the *Body-for-Life* Program Works." http//www.hussman.com/EAS/ Accessed 1/21/01.

3 Volek, J. and A. Campbell. "Trade Your Belly for Biceps." *Men's Health.* 2007. November. pp. 134-138.

4 Vogel, R.A. et al., "Effect of a single high-fat meal on an endothelial function in healthy subjects." *American Journal of Cardiology.* 79(3): 350-354. 1997.

5 Hussman, J., "Why the *Body-for-Life* Program Works." http//www.hussman.com/EAS/ Accessed 1/21/01.

6 Ibid.

7 Stoppani, J. and J. Wuebben, "Spot On Diet." *Muscle & Fitness. 2006; 68(6): 142.*

8 American College of Sports Medicine. Proper and improper weight loss programs. *Medical Science Sports Exercise.* 1983; 15: 534-539.

9 Ballor, D.L. et al., "Resistance weight training during caloric restriction enhances lean body weight maintenance." *American Journal of Clinical Nutrition.* 1988; 47:19-25.

10 Campbell, T.C. and Thomas Campbell, *The China Study.* Ben Bella Books. 2006. (p. 59-61)

11 Hyman, M. and Mark Liponis, *Ultra Prevention.* Scribner. 2006.

12 Weise, E., "Is it More Moral to be a Vegetarian?" *USA Today.* Life (p. 7D) 12-10-2009.

13 Perricone, N., *The Perricone Weight Loss Diet.* Ballantine Books. 2005. (p. 46)

14 Campbell, T.C. and Thomas Campbell, *The China Study.* Ben Bella Books. 2006. (p. 58)

15 Atkins, R.C., *Dr. Atkins New Diet Revolution.* Avon Books, Harper Collins 2002. (p. 51)

16 Ibid. (p. 314)

17 Cleve, T.L., *Saccharine Disease: The Master Disease of Our Time.* Keats Publishing. 1975.

18 Willet, W. et al., "A Prospective Study of Dietary Glycemic Load, Carbohydrate Intake and Risk of Coronary Heart Disease in U.S. Women." *American Journal of Clinical Nutrition.*

19 Campbell, A. "The Cure for Diabetes." *Men's Health.* 2006. December. pp. 136-142.

20 Hyman, M., *Ultrametabolism.* Scribner. 2006. (p. 43)

21 Chandalia, M. et al., "Beneficial Effects of High Fiber Intake in Patients with Type 2 Diabetes Mellitus." *New England Journal of Medicine.* 342, 2000: 1392-1398.

22 Hu, F.B. et al., "Frequent Nut Consumption and Coronary Heart Disease in Women: Prospective Cohort Study." *British Medical Journal.* 317 (7169) 1998. 1341-1345.

23 Rosenthal, E., "In Europe it's fish oil after heart attacks, but not in the U.S." *New York Times.* 2006. Oct. 3

24 Perricone, N. *The Perricone Weight Loss Diet.* Ballantine Books. 2005. (pp. 95-96)

25 Hyman, M., *Ultrametabolism.* Scribner. 2006. (p. 41).

26 Volek, J. and A. Campbell. "Trade Your Belly for Biceps." *Men's Health.* 2007. November. pp. 134-138.

27 Willett, W.C. et al., "Intake of Trans Fatty Acids and Risk of Coronary Heart Disease in Women." *Lancet.* 341 (8845) 1993. (pp. 581-585)

28 DeCastro, J.M., "The time of day and food intake influences overall intake in humans." *Journal of Nutrition.* Jan. 2004; 134(1): 104-111.

29 Ludwig, D., "High glycemic index foods, overeating and obesity." *Pediatrics.* 1999; 102(3): 26.

30 Antonio, J. and J. Stout., *Sports Supplements.* Lippincott Williams and Wilkins. 2001. (p. 211).

31 Zuckerbrot, T., "The Science of Weight Loss." *Men's Fitness.* May 2006. (p. 28)

Chapter 7: The Connect With Nature Weight Loss Solution

1 Thompson, D., *Medicine & Science in Sports & Exercise.* May 2004. (p. 911-914)

2 Chopra, D. and D. Simon, *Training the Mind, Healing the Body.* (Audio series). Nightingale-Conant. 1997.

3 Campbell, T.C. and Thomas Campbell, *The China Study.* Ben Bella Books. 2006. (p. 92)

4 Perricone, N., *The Perricone Weight Loss Diet.* Ballantine Books. 2005. (p. 57).

5 Campbell, T.C. and Thomas Campbell, *The China Study.* Ben Bella Books. 2006. (p. 143)

Chapter 8: The Power of Purpose

1 Dyer, W., *It's Never Too Crowded Along the Extra Mile: My Top 10 Secrets for Success & Inner Peace.* Hay House. 2001.
2 Jung, C., *Synchronicity: An Acausal Connecting Principle.* Princeton University Press. 1973.
3 Chopra, D., *The Spontaneous Fulfillment of Desire.* Random House. 2003. (Audio).
4 Chpra, D., *Ageless Body — Timeless Mind.* Crown Publishing Group. 1994. (p. 86)
5 Owen, F., "Running From Addiction." *Maxim.* September, 2008. (pp. 64-66)
6 Deitz, W.H., "Health consequences of obesity in youth: childhood predictors of adult disease." *Pediatrics.* 101 (1998): 518-525.
.

Chapter 9: Workout Plans

1 Chopra, D. and D. Simon, *Training the Mind, Healing the Body.* (Audio series). Nightingale-Conant. 1997.
2 Ibid.

Chapter 10: Warming Up and Cooling Down

1 Whitmarsh, B., *Mind and Muscle: Psyche Up, Build Up.* Human Kinetics. 2001.
2 Ibid.
3 Kristal, A. et al., "Yoga practice is associated with attenuated weight gain in healthy, middle-aged men and women." *Alternative Therapy Health Med.* 2005; 11(4): 28-33.
4 Robbins, A., *Ultimate Power: The New Science of Personal Achievement.* Simon and Schuster. 1997.
5 Devereau, G., *Dynamic Yoga: The Ultimate Workout That Chills Your Mind As It Changes Your Body.* Thorsons GBR. 1999.
6 Ibid.
7 Ibid.
8 Kraftsow, G., *Yoga for Wellness: Healing With The Timeless Teachings of Viniyoga.* Viking Penguin. 1999.

Chapter 11: Lockdown: The 20-Minute Total Body Workout

1 Hussman, J., "Why the *Body-for-Life* Program Works." http//www.hussman.com/EAS/p3. Accessed 1/21/01.
2 Covey, S.R., *The 7 Habits of Highly Effective People: Powerful Lessons in Personal Change.* Simon and Schuster. 1990.

Chapter 12: Walk in Nature Workouts

1 Chopra, D. and D. Simon, *Training the Mind, Healing the Body.* (Audio series). Nightingale-Conant. 1997.
2 Ibid.
3 Ibid.
4 Ibid
5 Ibid.

Chapter 14: The Convict's Mean and Lean Workouts

1 Kennedy, D., "Guerrilla Cardio," *Muscle Media* magazine, October 2001
2 Hyman, M. and M. Liponis, *Ultraprevention.* Scribner. 2003.
3 Hussman, J., "Why the *Body-for-Life* Program Works.*" http//www.hussman.com/EAS/ Accessed 1/21/01.
4 Phillips, B., *Sports Supplement Review.* Mile High Publishing. 1999. (p. 280)
5 Quill, S., Muscle Bulletion, *Men's Health.* Jan/Feb 2006 (p.136)

Chapter 15: Pay It Forward

1 Dyer, W., *The Power of Intention: Learning to Co-Create Your World Your Way.* (Audio) Hay House. 2004.
2 Ibid.
3 Frankl, V., *Man's Search for Meaning: An Introduction to Logotherapy.* Buckaneer Press. 1973

Principles of Grace — A Sneak Preview

1 Chopra, D. and D. Simon, *Training the Mind, Healing the Body.* (Audio series). Nightingale-Conant. 1997.
2 Maslow, A., *The Farthest Reaches of Human Nature.* Viking Penguin. 1993.
3 Covey, S.R., *The 7 Habits of Highly Effective People: Powerful Lessons in Personal Change.* Simon and Schuster. 1990.
4 Chopra, D., *The Spontaneous Fulfillment of Desire.* (Audio) Random House. 2003.
5 Dyer, W., *The Power of Intention: Learning to Co-create Your World Your Way.* (Audio). Hay House. 2004.
6 Ibid.
7 Dyer, W., *It's Never Too Crowded Along the Extra Mile: My Top 10 Secrets for Success & Inner Peace.* Hay House. 2001.

ABOUT THE AUTHOR

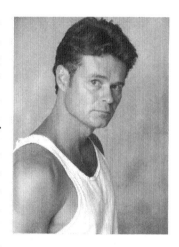

J. Barrett Hawkins is an entrepreneur and a writer. In 1985, at the age of 22, he opened a retail clothing store named Just Sweats. Over the next few years the company grew to become a thriving 22-store chain in the states of Ohio and Kentucky. In 1991, Hawkins was tried and convicted of insurance fraud (a crime he committed) and conspiracy to commit murder (a crime he did not knowingly or intentionally commit) and was sentenced to life in prison. There he read Viktor Frankl's classic book, *Man's Search for Meaning*, which encouraged him to find meaning in his suffering and to become aware of what he longed for in the depths of his heart. Hawkins' heart was the heart of a businessman, and what he longed for was an opportunity to prove to his son and to the victim's family that he was not the type of person who could knowingly be involved in the killing of a fellow human being. He hoped that he might be able to accomplish that objective by developing a business that would contribute to society in some meaningful way.

From his prison cell, Hawkins spent the next five years researching and developing two very different business concepts. The first, Hooked On Health, is an entirely new kind of medical establishment called a "transformation center," designed to guide patients through every stage of a health care transformation. The second, The Awakening Grace Learning Center, is a middle school/computer learning center hybrid that will provide educational opportunities for at-risk children.

As a means of communicating his visions, Hawkins devoted an additional five years to writing two books. One, titled *Penitentiary Fitness: The Amazing Weight Loss Formula,* encourages readers to pursue optimal health through proper nutrition and never-before-seen "convict workouts." The other, *Principles of Grace: The Teachings of the Medicine Man,* proposes that every human being was born with a specific purpose in life, and inspires readers to find that purpose through their deepest passions and service to others.

The author's third book, *The Entrepreneurs' Challenge*, is autobiographical in nature. In it Hawkins talks about the insurance fraud for the very first time. However, this book is not about crime; it is about the author's quest for redemption. *The Entrepreneurs' Challenge* is an e-series that can be purchased through the author's website: www.JBarrettHawkins.com.

AUTHOR'S WEBSITE

www.JBarrettHawkins.com

The author's website is a valuable resource for individuals who aspire to achieve optimal health, lose weight, or develop a lean, muscular physique.

I am constantly researching all areas of personal growth, in particular those dealing with health promotion, weight loss, purpose in life, and human intuition, and seek outstanding examples to share with my readers. You can download free sample chapters from all of my books or sign up for my free monthly syndicated column: *Ask Penitentiary Fitness.* I welcome you to visit the website and share your experiences with the ideas presented in this book. You can even send me information that you feel would be of interest to others who are actively pursuing personal growth.

I love hearing from readers. Anyone wanting to contact me may do so at:

info@darkplanetpublishing.com
— or —
info@penfit.com
My prison address is available at my website.

—Also by J. Barrett Hawkins —

THE DIRTY NASTY TRUTH

J. Barrett Hawkins is a member of a juvenile delinquency/crime prevention organization named CROP, where at-risk youths are brought into Donovan State Prison in San Diego to hear criminals speak about crime, gangs, self-esteem, and prison life. In this 70-minute audio book, Hawkins describes three true crime stories and a program that will assist parents in developing their child's self-esteem.

First, Hawkins discusses his involvement in a million-dollar insurance fraud that he believed would be a victimless, white-collar crime, and explains how that scheme was directly responsible for the murder of an innocent man. You will learn that there is no such thing as a victimless crime. Hawkins also talks about his attempted suicide. This segment concludes with an illuminating discussion on the "near death experience." You'll find convincing scientific evidence that the soul lives on following the body's death.

Next, Hawkins relates the story of 16-year-old gang member Diego Jones, who is serving 50 years to life for a double homicide. Jones's gut-wrenching story revolves around a deadly shootout between rival gang members.

The third true crime story is that of Joe Jackson, who the FBI dubbed "The Gentleman Bank Robber." Jackson's is a classic "gateway" drug story in that alcohol and marijuana use became the gateway to a serious cocaine addiction. In order to get the money needed to pay for the drugs, Jackson committed a series of bank robberies.

The stories of Jones and Jackson serve as a prelude to a discussion on developing self-esteem. In the final part of *The Dirty Nasty Truth* you will learn that the primary reason that teenagers join gangs, use drugs, or engage in criminal behavior is because they suffer from low self-esteem. Hawkins shares insights from his 10-year study of developing self-esteem, discovering purpose in life, and fulfilling one's dreams. The audio book concludes with Hawkins describing the qualities, behaviors, and success secrets of some of the world's top achievers.

Quick Order Form

Telephone Orders: Call (760) 747-2734. Have your credit card ready.
E-mail Orders: Store@DarkPlanetPublishing.com
Postal Orders: Dark Planet Publishing
1256 Industrial Ave.
Escondido, CA 92029

Please send the following books or CDs:

	Price	Quantity	Costs
Penitentiary Fitness soft cover book	$19.95		
Principles of Grace soft cover book	$19.95		
The Dirty Nasty Truth audio CD	$14.00		
The Amazing Weight Loss Formula audio CD	$14.00		
Penitentiary Fitness T-shirt	$20.00		
Penitentiary Fitness tank top	$20.00		
Penitentiary Fitness sweatshirt	$40.00		
Shipping & Handling			
Sales Tax			
TOTAL COSTS			

Sales tax: Please add 8.25% for products shipped to California addresses
Shipping & Handling: $4.95 for the first book or CD, and $2.00 for each additional product. The products will be mailed media rate. If you need speedier delivery, contact us to discuss other options.

Payment: ☐ Check ☐ Credit Card

☐ VISA ☐ MASTERCARD

Card number: _____
Name on Card: _____
Expiration Date: _____

Shipping Information: _____
Name: _____
Address: _____
City: _____ **State:** ____ **Zip:** _____
Telephone: _____
E-mail address: _____

Made in the USA
Charleston, SC
25 July 2011